glamour gurlz

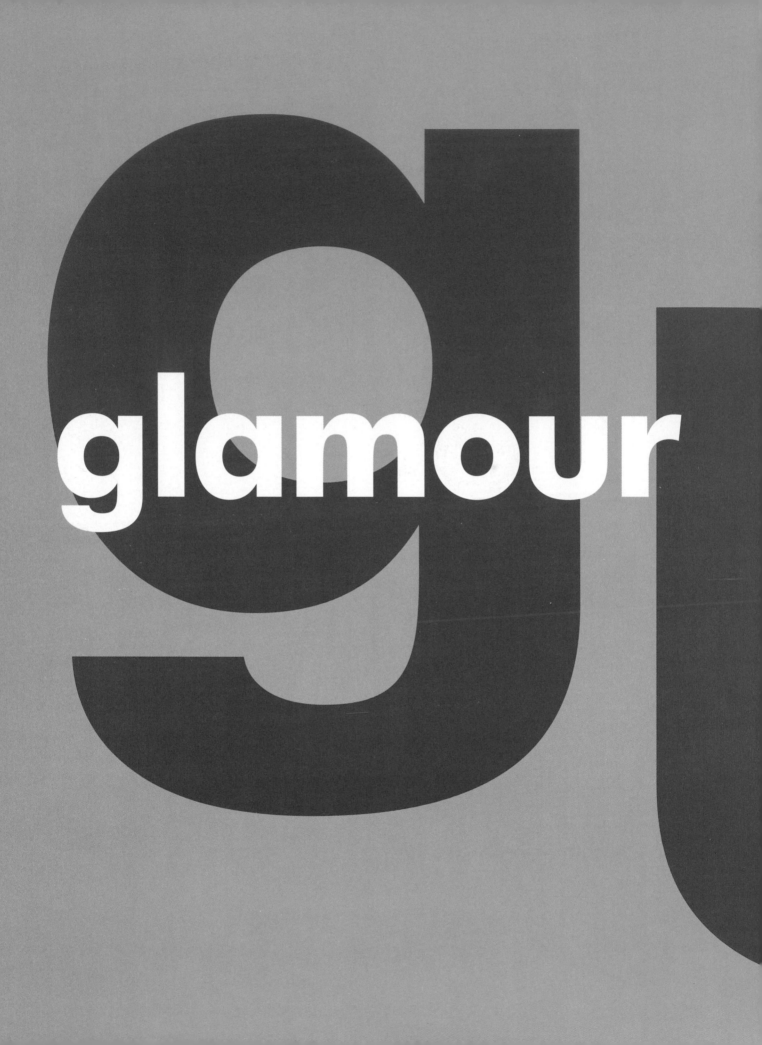

glamour

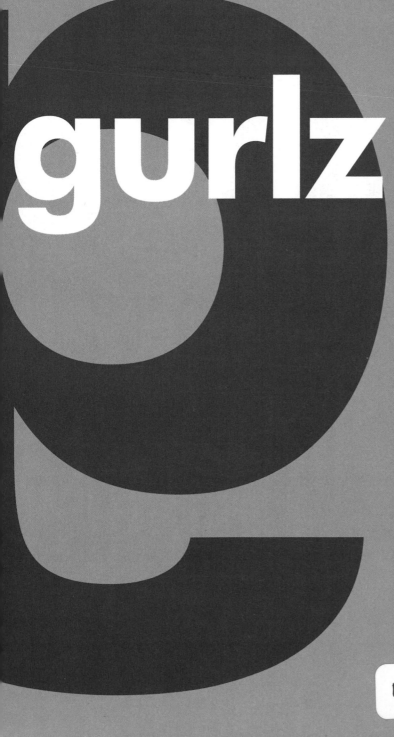

gurlz

**The Ultimate Step-by-Step
Guide to Great Makeup
and Gurl Smarts**

Joanna Schlip

**Clarkson Potter/Publishers
New York**

The truth is, no matter put on or how beautiful outside . . . nothing com important than—feeling

how much makeup you you appear on the pares to—or is more beautiful on the inside.

Joanna Schlip

contents

INTRODUCTION 9

techniques

the glamour gurlz

tricks of the trade

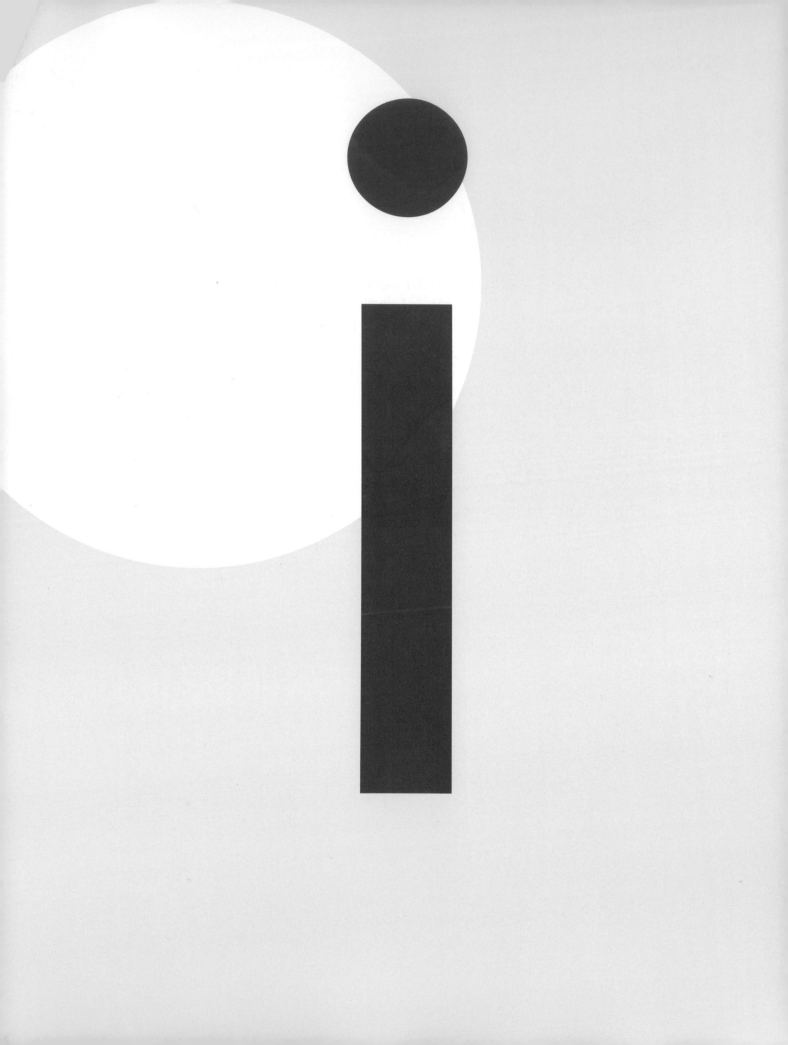

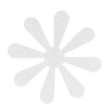

Introduction

A little more than two years ago, amid the hustle and bustle of my career as a professional makeup artist, a cup of scalding tea changed everything. I never imagined that something so common could affect my fun and busy life.

But that's exactly what happened. One abrupt stop in my car sent my take-out container of hot tea flying and sent me to the skin center with a third of my face covered in second- and third-degree burns.

After many treatments, I was left with raw, red wounds and a great deal of scar tissue. I couldn't believe it! I found it unbearable to look at myself and felt extremely self-conscious working so closely with the beautiful models and celebrities who had become part of my daily routine.

But more disturbing was how this burn changed me on the *inside*. I had always thought of myself as a strong, confident woman. But all those feelings seemed to disappear the second I saw myself in the mirror; suddenly all of the confidence I'd developed over the years was gone! It was as if I had become my young, insecure teen self all over again.

I didn't want to be stared at.

I didn't want to stand out.

I didn't want to have to tell the story over and over again.

These facial burns, the scarring, and the long, very public process of my healing forced me to reevaluate myself. Could it be that all of that adult confidence I felt was really just confidence in the way I *looked?* I came to realize that, from an early age, many of the ideas I had about beauty—and even about being accepted by others—were far more wrapped up in *how I looked* than in *who I had become*. I also realized that when the accident happened, my initial concerns weren't about my health, but more about what had happened to my appearance—and what might happen to my career in the beauty industry.

Can you imagine? I worried that, no matter how good I am at what I do, people would not want to work with me if they didn't find me pretty!

The moment I came to this realization . . . this book was born.

I knew I had to get out there and do what I loved: makeup. I discovered that facing my fears head-on was the best medicine for everything that was making me feel bad . . . and, that if *I* could do it, I could teach young Gurlz to do the same.

I wrote *Glamour Gurlz* to help teens understand that happiness is directly related to feeling strong and confident in your *abilities*, not just in how you look. To develop this sense of confidence with makeup, school, and anything else, I encourage all Gurlz to trust their instincts.

If you love makeup, you've picked up the right book. As a makeup artist who's created looks for every major fashion magazine you've read (and many others you'll read as your look develops), I'll give you the secret 4-1-1 on how any Gurl can live out her Glamour Gurl fantasy. The trick? Getting the right *attitude:* Makeup is fun, but it's just an *accessory.*

Makeup is *not* your whole identity. In fact, just as you have different moods, you can also have more than one side to your personality, but it's still *you,* just another expression of you. What do I mean? Using different makeup looks to express different sides of you is like having different friends from different groups, different feelings, different hobbies depending on where you are and whom you're with. Just flip through and you'll figure out which look or combination of looks you want to try!

In the following pages you'll see how a *professional makeup artist* can create different looks that make Gurlz feel fun, confident, and pretty. I'll also show you step by step how you can create your own version of this look. But remember that real beauty and confidence are already inside you.

So, are you ready to discover your inner Glamour Gurl?

Me and my nieces,
Brit and Katie

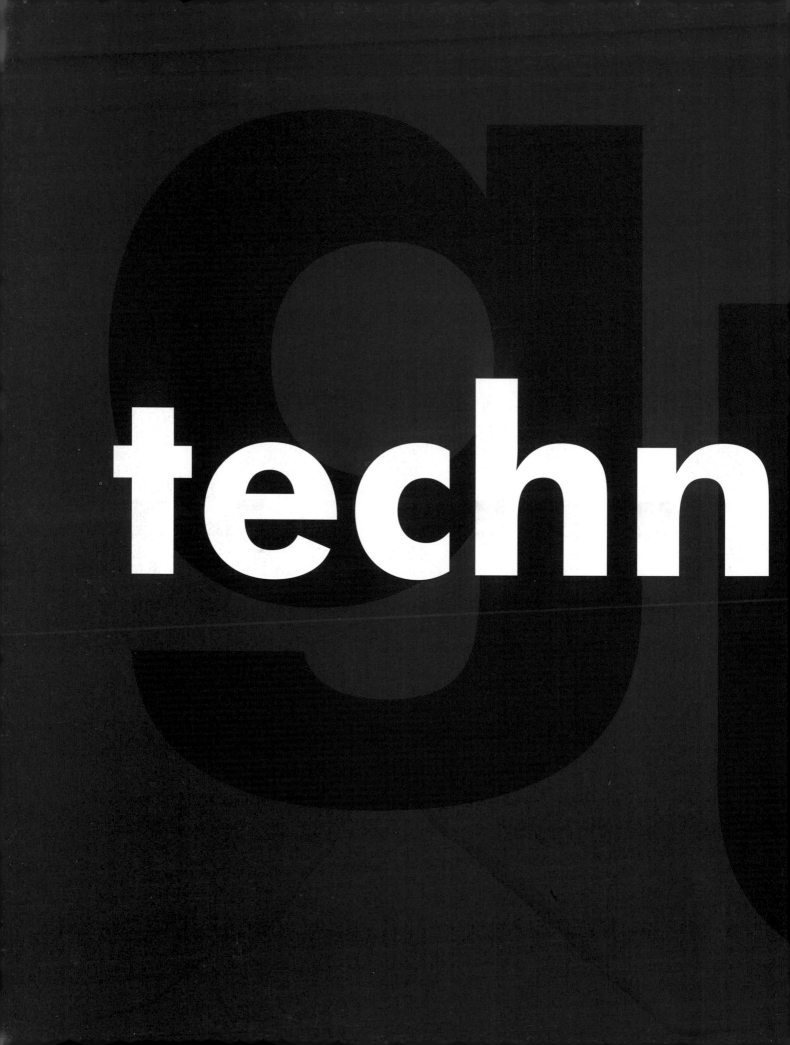

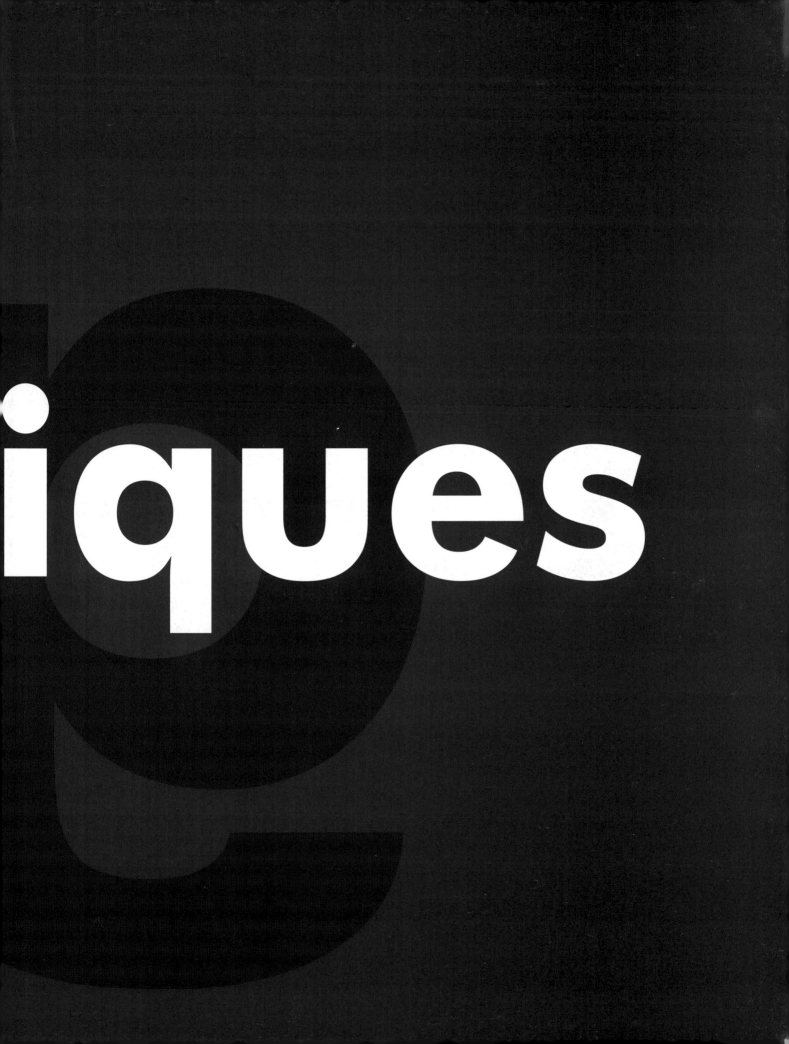

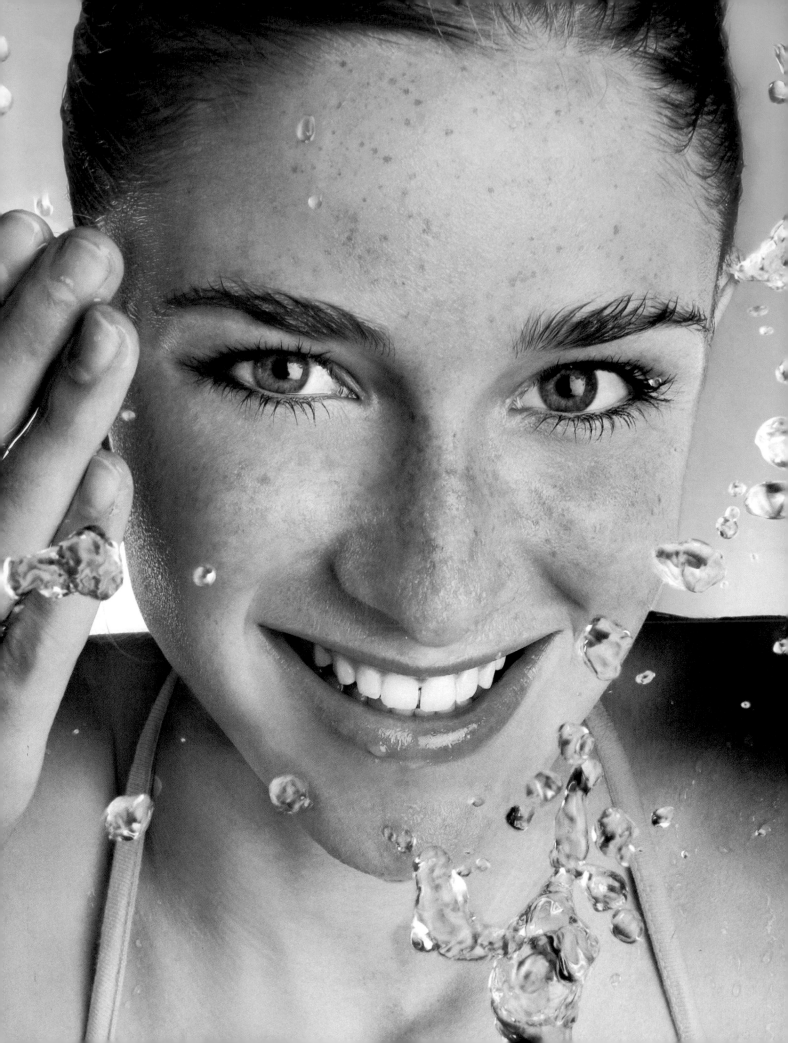

Complexion Perfection!

What skin type am I?

In order to learn how to care for your skin, you must first identify what skin type you have:

DRY SKIN

If your skin tends to get flaky or feel tight, then you are probably *dry*.

NORMAL SKIN

Normal skin doesn't flake or feel tight on a regular basis. Normal skin does tend to look shiny after lunchtime, around 2 pm.

OILY SKIN

Do you get shiny after breakfast, around 10 am? If so, you probably have *oily* skin.

SENSITIVE SKIN

Not sure if your skin is sensitive? Use two fingers to press down on your cheeks and hold them there for a few seconds. If you have a bright red mark, then your skin is *sensitive*.

COMBINATION SKIN

Skin that does not fit squarely into one category and includes characteristics from two or more skin types is *combination*. For example, it's common for teen Gurlz to have normal skin with an oilier *T-zone*—the area of your forehead and down your nose to your chin.

Why does skin type matter? Because different skin requires different steps to cleanse and prepare prior to applying makeup. When I prep skin, I look at the overall appearance to determine the skin type and area types. Does she have oily skin? Or just an oily T-zone? Once I understand the skin I'm working with, then I tackle any "problems" I see. For example, when I see *dry* skin, I prep the skin for makeup by moisturizing. This allows the makeup to apply more smoothly and avoids streaking. *Oily* skin lets me know that I should skip the moisturizer step and instead apply a non-comedogenic tinted moisturizer with sunblock, followed by a light dusting of powder to absorb any oil that comes up throughout the day. For *combination* skin I do the same, but only powder the areas that tend to get oily, like the T-zone. Finally, if I notice that a Gurl has *sensitive* skin, I make a point of using only *hypoallergenic* products on her and avoiding anything that might contain perfume. Remember, when you have sensitive skin, almost anything can cause a red reaction!

Skincare Basics in Three Steps: Cleanse, Tone, Hydrate

CLEANSE

Professionals advise Gurlz to cleanse twice, two times a day. Meaning, wash your face once to clear away makeup, and then wash again to actually clean your skin of bacteria and dirt. Cleanse your skin this way twice a day, both morning and night, with a cleansing product that matches your skin type.

TONE

Toners are used to balance your skin. They hydrate the skin and tighten your pores.

HYDRATE

Use a light moisturizer to hydrate the skin. Pick one designed for your skin type and use it every day.

Acne Alert!

Acne is a condition that's common to teen skin. Whatever the degree, spots should be treated with products designed to calm acne inflammation (redness) and combat young skin's tendency to overproduce oil. Serious acne should be treated by a dermatologist.

UNDER COVER

Operation: Cover Up

Most **foundation** is too heavy for teen skin, which makes **tinted moisturizer** the perfect cover-up! If you feel like you need a little more coverage in some areas or on spots, use your concealer. To apply tinted moisturizer, use a brush, a sponge, or *clean* fingers.

Concealer should be blended under the eyes until it sets. Tap-tap-tap with your ring finger until your concealer doesn't have hard edges, but still covers up darkness.

When it comes to concealer and tinted moisturizer, always choose light and non-comedogenic products that won't clog your pores.

When you're concealing under the eyes, your concealer should be one shade lighter for pale skin and two shades lighter for darker skin. On the other hand, when covering a pimple, your concealer should match your skin almost exactly. You can mix your concealer with tinted moisturizer to get the perfect color for pimple coverage. Use a **tiny brush** for precise coverage. Don't forget to set it with powder.

Use **face/translucent powder** to set your tinted moisturizer and concealer. A **soft fluffy puff** is your best loose powder tool. Dip the puff gently, shake off the excess, rub a little in your palm and then press your powder puff all over to set your tinted moisturizer. Wash your powder puffs once a week with soap and warm water.

SPOT TREAT!

If you don't have acne all over, don't use acne products all over. Far too often healthy or normal skin becomes dried out when Gurlz overuse acne products in areas of the skin that never break out. This forms a layer of dead skin cells that block the normal release of oil and cause more pimples!

The most important rule when treating acne is IF IT'S INFLAMED STAY AWAY! DO NOT PICK, POKE, SQUEEZE, or SCRATCH. Doing any of this can cause a spot's pocket of bacteria to burst and empty onto the skin around it, causing more pimples to develop and possibly an infection.

Sun Smartz

Use sun protection and use it every day! When choosing a sun product, look at the bottle: Each SPF—SPF 8, 10, or 45—represents how many times longer the product will protect you from the sun than your natural protection would. In other words, a product with SPF 10 will provide protection for ten times longer than you could normally be in the sun before turning red and then burning. So if your skin naturally burns in ten minutes, applying SPF 10 will allow you to be in the sun for 100 minutes (10 minutes $\times$ SPF 10) before burning. If you plan on being out in the sun longer than that, you'll have to reapply, or you won't be protected! Sunscreens must be applied a half hour before going out into the sun and reapplied throughout the day. Don't forget, even going to and from school exposes you to the sun long enough to cause sun damage.

To avoid breakouts, choose a sunblock that is *non-comedogenic*. Products of this type are designed not to block pores.

Want to skip a step? Choose a non-comedogenic moisturizer or tinted moisturizer that *includes* sunblock for daytime. Use a regular moisturizer for nighttime.

BLUSH ON!

You can choose a powder, crème, or gel blush. To apply, smile and find the "apple" of your cheek—that's the round circle your cheek makes when you smile. If you choose a powder, pick up your *round* brush and dab the brush into the powder. Now shake off the brush to remove excess product and avoid streaking when you apply. Smile and swirl your brush around the apples of your cheeks in a circular motion and flick the brush up lightly toward your ears. That way you're both highlighting *and* defining your cheek, at the same time.

Crème, gel, or stain blushes are also awesome! They're easy to use *and* can double as a crème eyeshadow or lip color. To apply, smile . . . and use your fingers to rub a little on the apples of your cheeks. Blend up and voilà! You've got a creamy, glowing complexion.

LIP APPEAL

If your lip gloss has a brush or foam wand, you're all set. But if your lip gloss comes in a pot, consider getting a lip brush for a perfect application every time—and to avoid wiping sticky gloss on your jeans . . .

If you're going for a dramatic lip, start by filling in the center of your lips with a lip gloss that has a lot of color pigment in it—meaning, the *less sheer* lip gloss. Then grab a lip liner that's nearly the same color as the lip gloss and draw a perfect edge around your lips. Blend the two together. Now you have that perfect glamour pout!

Obvious lip liner is *so last millennium.* In other words, lip liner is a tool to be used only when the look calls for more drama. When you do use it, keep your liner the same color as your lip gloss. Never too dark!

EYE GOT IT!

Eye shadow is all about building up the look of your eyes, making them look more *defined.* Start with less eye shadow than you think you need, evaluate in the mirror, and add more color as you see fit. You'll have flawless eyes in no time, and never have to clean off for a redo!

Eyeliner can be a touchy subject because some people *love* their eyeliner, even if the people around them think it's *way too much.* Your eyeliner should always be flattering, not scary. After all, you want to show your *eyes,* not your *liner!* If you prefer to use a liquid eyeliner during the day, soften the edge and the overall look by rubbing a very small amount of black or another matching color of eye shadow along the line. It's also fun to smudge together two different shades of eyeliner and shadow, like blue shimmer shadow over black eyeliner.

Eyelash curlers allow you to create a soft, finished eyelash look. Only curl your top lashes. Apply mascara *after* you curl, then follow with a **lash comb** to un-clump your mascara. Remember, all mascara, no matter how expensive, will get clumpy from time to time. A few sweeps with your lash comb will keep that fringe fluttering!

I like using black mascara for every look, because I think it gives you a clean look with way more bang for your mascara buck! Use waterproof mascara if you plan to play sports, work out, or if you might be walking in the rain. Otherwise, raccoon eyes, Gurl . . .

PLUCK IT!

The first time you pluck your eyebrows, you may find it painful and difficult to get a nice, symmetrical eyebrow shape. Still want to try? Check out these tips.

NUMB IT!

If you find it painful to groom your brows, briefly apply ice or an over-the-counter pain reliever for gums on the area you'd like to pluck. But not in your eye!

GET IT!

Before you take out any hairs, get great tweezers. What makes a great pair of tweezers? Choose a pair that's thin enough on the end, or they won't pick up your hairs. Slanted tips are also good.

PLAN IT!

Create a grid that will be your plucking guide; that way you won't mess up. Your eyebrows should *start* directly above *where your eyes begin*. To check this, hold a Popsicle stick against your nose, lined up with where your inner eye begins; that's where your inner brow should *begin*. Do this for both eyes and then clean everything between these two lines.

Now line your stick up from the outside edge of your nostril to the outside corner where your eye ends, extending all the way to the outside edge of your eyebrow. That's where the eyebrow should end.

Pick up your Popsicle stick one last time. Look straight ahead and line the stick up from the outside edge of your nostril, to your pupil (the black dot in the middle of your eyeball); that's where your arch should be. Take a white eyebrow pencil and white out all the hairs you plan to pluck in order to create this arch. Stand back and check that you like what you see. Remember, you shouldn't remove the natural shape of your brow, just the excess, or the hairs that need to go in order to enhance the shape.

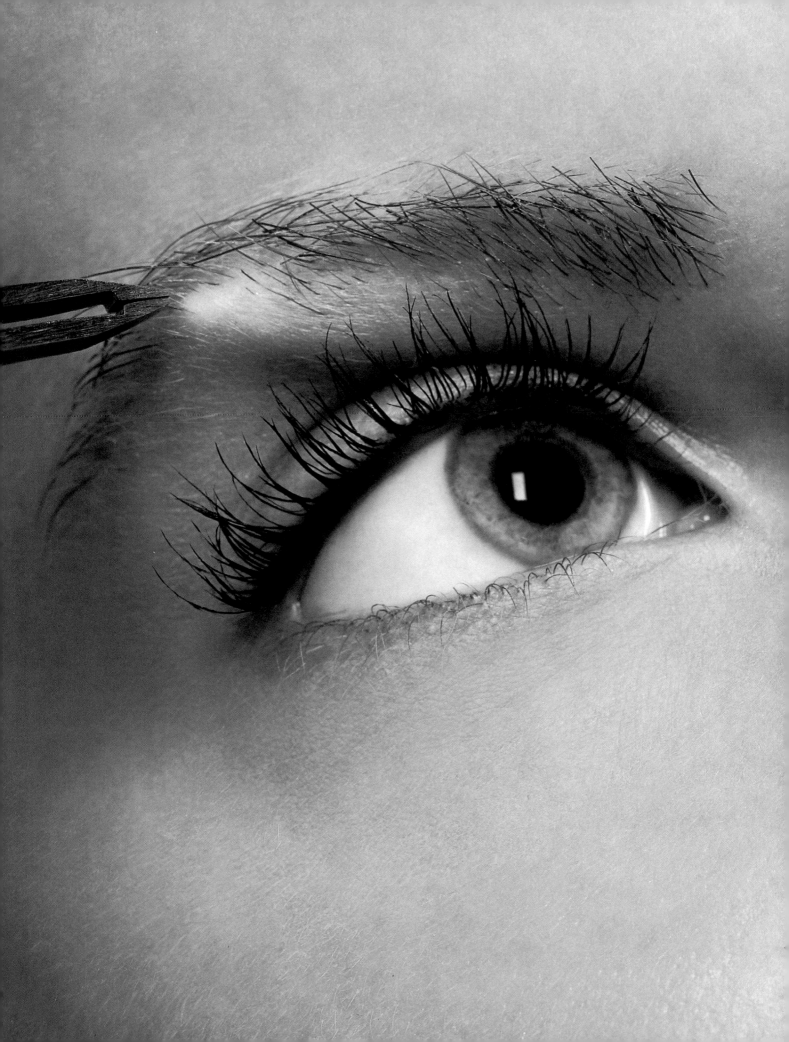

the glam

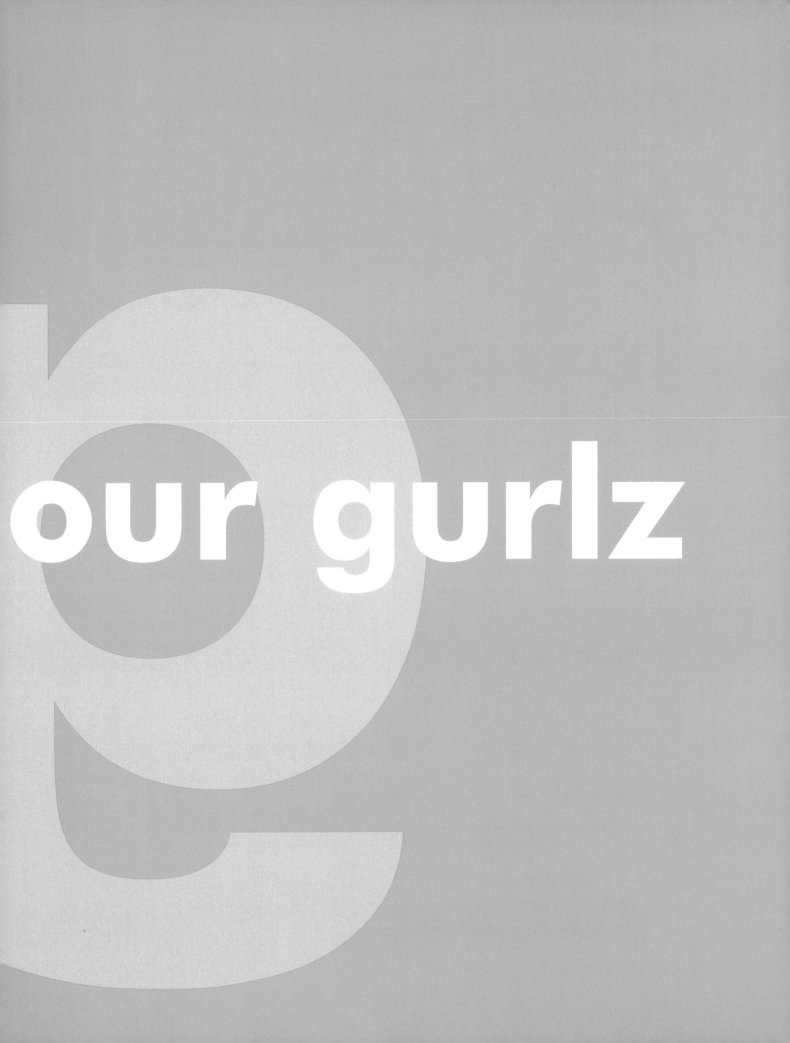

our gurlz

Amanda

Talk about ambition: This Gurl has drive. She wants to excel at everything: sports, school, and, most of all, expressing herself with great new looks.

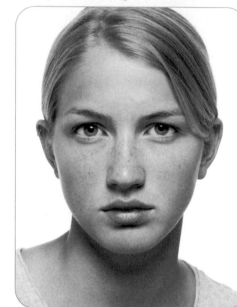

BEFORE: I brightened up under Amanda's eyes, evened out her skin tone, covered a few spots, and shaped her brows.

Tools
Toner
Moisturizer with SPF
Concealer
Face/Translucent powder
Pink powder blush
Sheer pink lip gloss
Brow gel
Blonde eyebrow pencil
Lash curler
Black mascara

Star LIGHT!

Get This Look

Step 1
Start with clean, prepped skin. Wash your face, then apply toner and a light moisturizer with SPF. Let the products soak into your skin for five minutes. Blot away any excess with a tissue.

Step 2
Apply concealer with your *ring* fingertip, that's the one next to your pinkie. Dab in the bottom and top inner corners of your eyes and below your eyes, out and over, or wherever you see blue, gray, or red. Blend down and out by tapping the concealer into place until there are no distinct lines. Rub any leftover concealer on any redness around your nostrils and on any spots.

Step 3
Set your concealer by lightly tapping translucent powder over it with a puff or a fluffy brush.

Step 4
Lightly dust the blush on the apples of your cheeks and blend out toward the ears.

Step 5
Sweep the gloss over your lips.

Step 6
Use the brush of your eyebrow gel to brush your eyebrows up and out. Fill in any gaps with the eyebrow pencil. Apply less than you think you should.

Step 7
Curl your lashes and apply one coat of mascara.

Why It's a Winner: This look calls for nothing on the eyelids, which keeps it clean and fresh.

What the Pros Say: "Look at this Gurl's eyes; you can tell that she's focusing on her future." —Tracy Bayne, photographer for Beyoncé Knowles

The Bigger Picture: Not all looks require eye makeup. The most striking "looks" always come from your eyes themselves!

The Look: Fresh, clean, and natural. Perfect for school, the beach, or any time you want to look put-together, without looking like you're *trying*.

ALL DOLLED UP

The Look: A clean, fun look that's perfect for a day at the mall with your Gurlz.

Tools
Toner
Tinted moisturizer with SPF
Concealer
Face/Translucent powder
Rose powder blush
Shimmery berry lip gloss
Brow gel
Blonde eyebrow pencil
White shimmer powder eye shadow
Lash curler
Black mascara

Get This Look

Step 1
Start with clean, prepped skin. Wash your face, then apply toner. Let the product soak into your skin for five minutes.

Step 2
Using clean hands, rub a tinted moisturizer with SPF on your face. Start at the center and blend out toward the ends of your face. Be sure to blend down your neck.

Step 3
Apply concealer with your *ring* fingertip, that's the one next to your pinkie. Dab in the bottom and top inner corners of your eyes and below your eyes, out and over, or wherever you see blue, gray, or red. Blend down and out by tapping the concealer into place until there are no distinct lines. Rub any leftover concealer on any redness around your nostrils and on any spots.

Step 4
Set your tinted moisturizer and concealer by lightly dusting powder over your face with a puff or a big fluffy brush.

Step 5
Dust the blush on the apples of your cheeks and blend out toward the ears.

Step 6
Apply the gloss with a lip brush.

Step 7
Use the brush of your eyebrow gel to brush your eyebrows up and out. Fill in any gaps with the eyebrow pencil. Apply less than you think you should.

Step 8
Using an eye shadow brush, dust the eye shadow from your lash line to your brow bone, keeping only the edges soft and blended. For this look, be sure to blend the shadow down into the corner of your eyes.

Step 9
Curl your lashes and apply one coat of mascara.

Why It's a Winner:

Applying white on the inside corners of your eyes really opens them up.

What the Pros Say:

"On the one hand, this is a classic, sweet, and clean look, but then her small earring gives the whole thing a bit of an edge." —James Charles, Director of New Faces, L.A. Models agency

The Bigger Picture:

Sometimes getting a look right takes time and practice. Don't be hard on yourself if you don't get it right the first time.

SCHLIPTIP ON TINTED MOISTURIZER: Moisturizers with skin-toned pigment in them are a great way to even out skin tone without looking like you're wearing a mask. But even within the world of tinted moisturizers, you'll find a variety of products that cover more or less depending on the amount of pigment they contain.

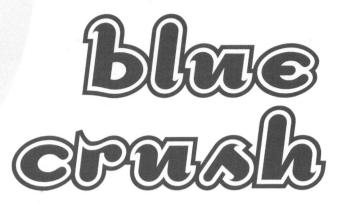

Tools
Toner
Tinted moisturizer with SPF
Concealer
Face/Translucent powder
Soft pink powder shimmer blush
Pink shimmer lip gloss
Brow gel
Blonde eyebrow pencil
Sky-blue powder eye shadow
Lash curler
Black mascara

blue crush

The Look: Sky-blue eyes, soft lips and cheeks . . .
ready for the game or the after party!

Get This Look

Step 1
Start with clean, prepped skin. Wash your face, then apply toner. Let the product soak into your skin for five minutes.

Step 2
Using clean hands, rub a tinted moisturizer with SPF on your face. Start at the center and blend out toward the ends of your face. Be sure to blend down your neck.

Step 3
Apply concealer with your *ring* fingertip, that's the one next to your pinkie. Dab in the bottom and top inner corners of your eyes and below your eyes, out and over, or wherever you see blue, gray, or red. Blend down and out by tapping the concealer into place until there are no distinct lines. Rub any leftover concealer on any redness around your nostrils and on any spots.

Step 4
Set your tinted moisturizer and concealer by lightly dusting powder over your face with a puff or a big fluffy brush.

Step 5
Lightly dust the blush on the apples of your cheeks and blend out toward the ears.

Step 6
Apply the gloss with a lip brush.

Step 7
Use the brush of your eyebrow gel to brush your eyebrows up and out. Fill in any gaps with the eyebrow pencil. Apply less than you think you should.

Step 8
Using an eye shadow brush, dip into your eye shadow and flick off the excess so you don't apply too much in one spot. Using a side-to-side motion, begin at your lash line and spread the powder all the way up to your brow bone.

Step 9
Curl your lashes and apply one coat of mascara.

Why It's a Winner: Sky blue opens up the eyes and lightly contrasts with the softer pink tones.

What the Pros Say: "Beauty comes from within. This Gurl's outer beauty reflects how beautiful she is on the inside!" —Andrew Matusik, photographer for Hilary Duff

The Bigger Picture: Like anything else in your life, makeup can sometimes be about taking risks. Wearing bright colors can be tough to pull off, but you never know what you can get away with until you try.

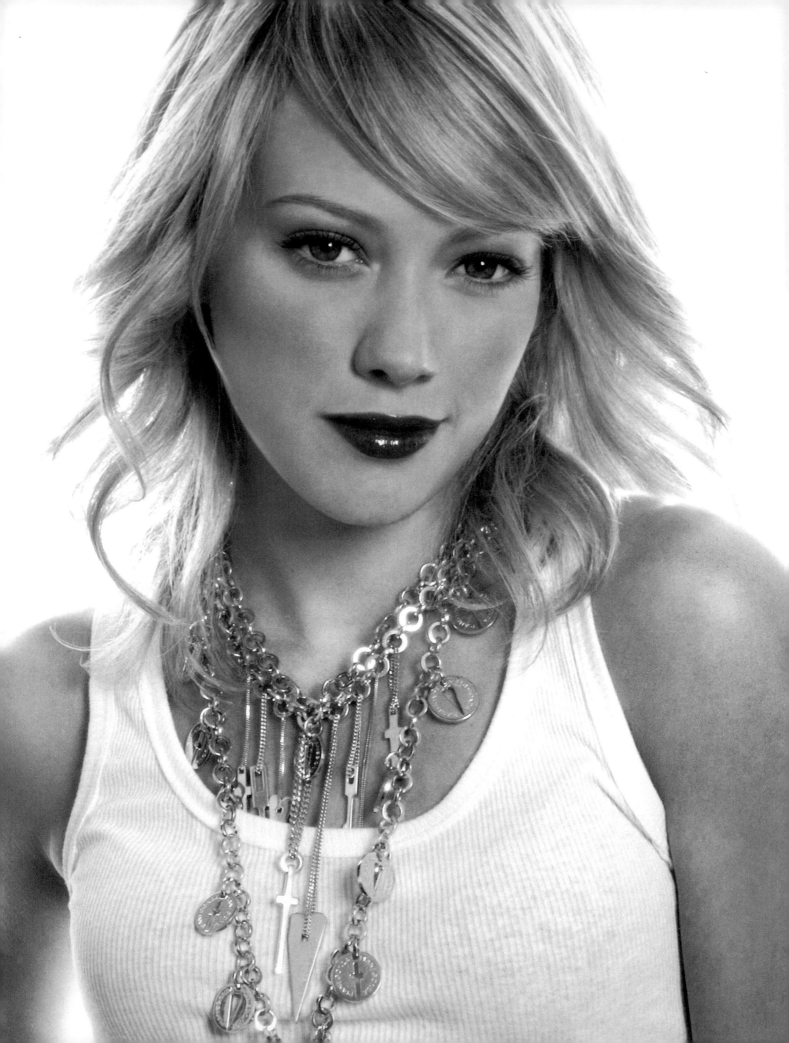

Hilary Duff

Actress, Singer, and Songwriter

I was blown away at how hard this Gurl works. Not only is she gorgeous and talented, but even though her schedule is to the max, she still found time to meet with me and talk about the importance of Gurlz feeling confident. When it's time to step up to the plate, this Gurl always does.

LIKE THIS LOOK? I gave this same look to Dashenka in "Candy Land" (page 44). I intensified Hilary's version by adding a warm brown pressed powder eye shadow up to the crease, followed by a cherry-red lip gloss.

Hilary Duff
Actress, Singer, and Songwriter

HILARY SAYS

"Real beauty is determined by the spirit: Kindness, generosity, and tolerance make people beautiful."

Like This Look? I gave this same look to Acia and Alia in "Double Dare" (page 36), except with Hilary, I skipped the black and smudged copper eye shadow along the top and bottom lash lines. I put a creamy apricot gloss on Hilary's lips.

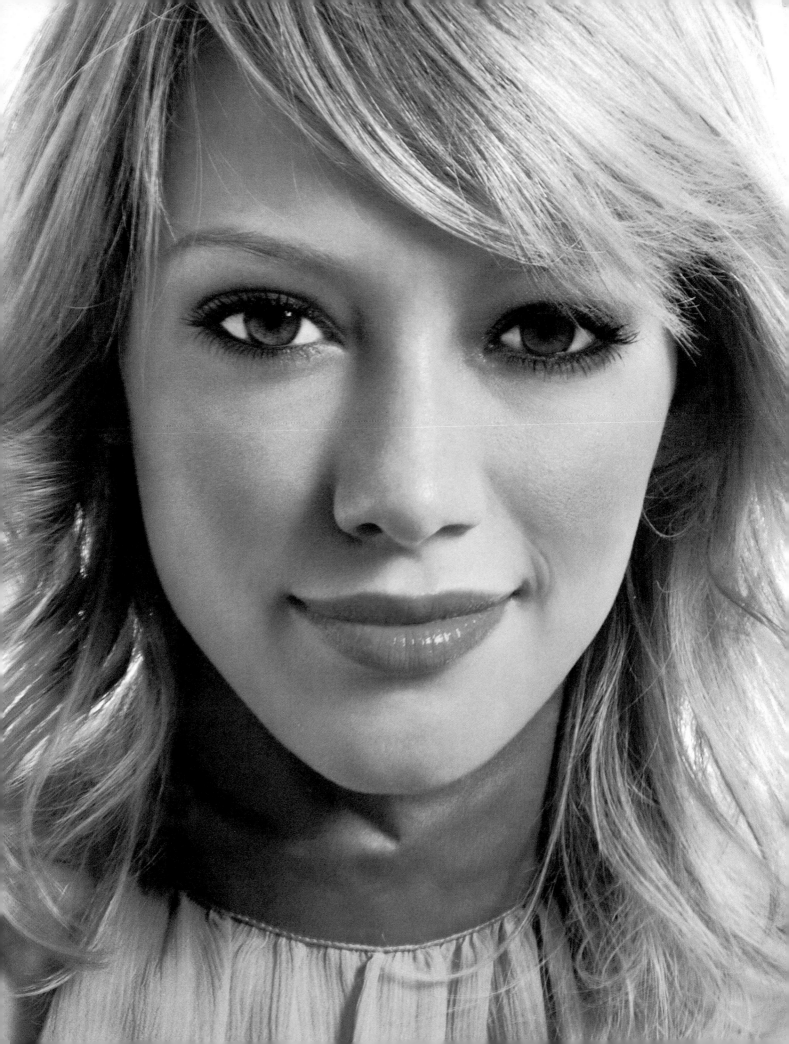

develop it!

Feeling confident is wonderful. But not if you're only feeling confident about your looks. If your feelings about yourself are too wrapped up in your image, does that mean a bad hair day will completely devastate you?

Real confidence comes from achievement. Find something you love to do; get really good at it and your confidence will grow!

The confidence you gain from doing something well will last a lifetime.

finding your groove

Finding your groove is not about doing what everyone else is doing. It's about listening to YOUR own inner rock star. Don't worry about what other people think; just do what you like doing and you'll find your groove!

Acia and Alia

MEET ACIA AND ALIA, identical twins. But here's the thing: Alia thinks Acia is beautiful, but is down on herself. And Acia thinks Alia is gorgeous, but feels bad about her own looks. So what's the deal? These Gurlz can see the beauty in each other's faces, just not in their own. Crazy, right?

All too often it's hard to see your own beauty. But even though you might not always feel like you're great, your real beauty is always there, just waiting for you to recognize it.

Like This Look?

It's the same as Double Dare on the next page. Instead of pink blush use a shimmer bronzer on the cheeks. Switch out the pink gloss for a caramel colored one. Using a black kohl pencil liner, only line above the eyes. No smudging! Keep the line thin and clean so you can really define your eyes.

DOUBLE DARE

BEFORE: Acia and Alia are both striking, but they tend to get dark circles around the eyes and spots that give them just a bit of uneven skin tone. I fixed these and also chose to shape their eyebrows.

The Look: Take the previous look and turn it on its head, by turning your eye technique upside down!

Tools
Toner
Tinted moisturizer with SPF
Concealer
Face/Translucent powder
Pink powder blush
Sheer pink lip gloss
Brow gel
Dark brown eyebrow pencil
Black kohl eyeliner pencil
Cotton swab
Lash curler
Black mascara

Get This Look

Step 1
Start with clean, prepped skin. Wash your face, then apply toner. Let the product soak into your skin for five minutes.

Step 2
Using clean hands, rub a tinted moisturizer with SPF on your face. Start at the center and blend out toward the ends of your face. Be sure to blend down your neck.

Step 3
Apply concealer with your *ring* fingertip, that's the one next to your pinkie. Dab in the bottom and top inner corners of your eyes and below your eyes, out and over, or wherever you see blue, gray, or red. Blend down and out by tapping the concealer into place until there are no distinct lines. Rub any leftover concealer on any redness around your nostrils and on any spots.

Step 4
Set your tinted moisturizer and concealer by lightly dusting powder over the face with a puff or a big fluffy brush.

Step 5
Wash the blush very lightly across your cheekbones and blend out.

Step 6
Use your lip brush to apply some lip gloss.

Step 7
Use the brush of your eyebrow gel to brush your eyebrows up and out. Fill in any gaps with the eyebrow pencil. Apply less than you think you should.

Step 8
Line all the way around the eye with eyeliner. Then line all around the *inside* of the eye and finish off by smudging the liner with a clean shadow brush or a cotton swab.

Step 9
Curl your lashes and apply *two* coats of mascara.

Why It's a Winner: This is a fresh look that is still cool enough for going out at night.

What the Pros Say: "These Gurlz are strong. You can see it in their attitudes and body language. This is a very powerful image." —Luc Brinker, model agent for Wilhelmina Models

The Bigger Picture: Simply changing how much or where you line your eyes can make a huge difference in how you look. Ever think about what other small changes—in attitude, schedule, and friends—can make a difference to your *whole life*?

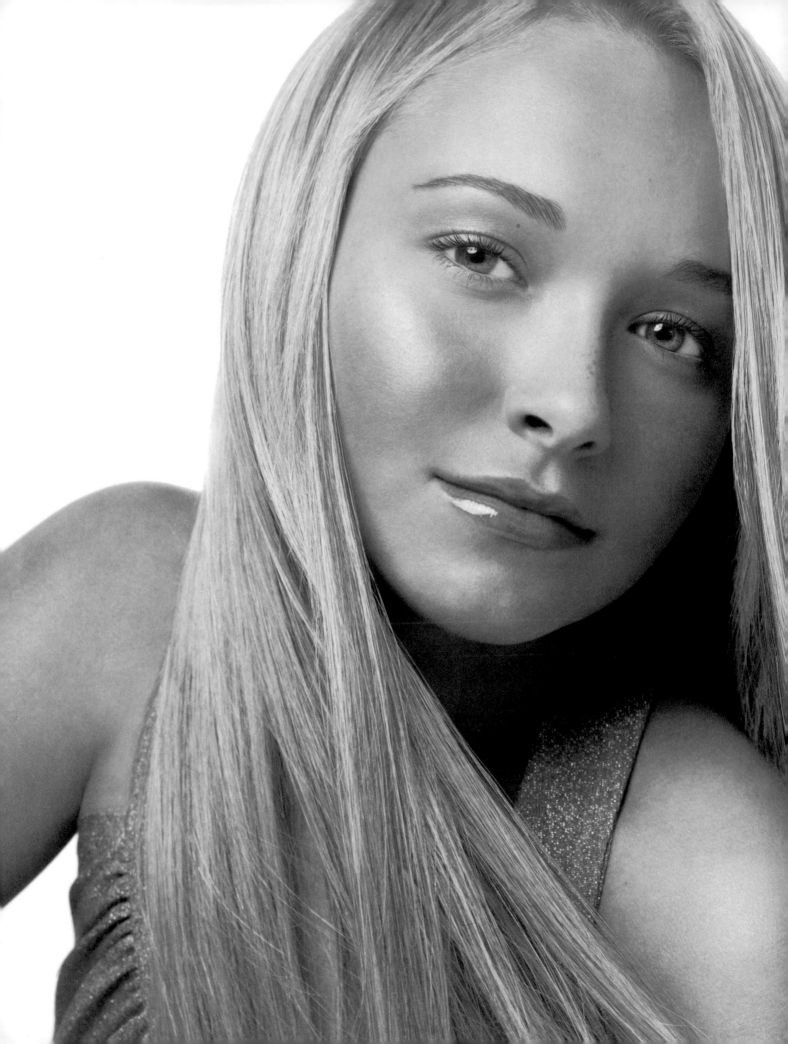

Hayden Panettiere
Actress and Singer

Hayden is one gorgeous Gurl who is not concerned with what other people think. She looks ahead, not to the side to see what others are doing. She's her own person in every beautiful way!

LIKE THIS LOOK? I gave this same look to Caitlin in "Prom Princess" (page 92). Notice how Hayden's eye shadow is just on her *top* lid, while Caitlin wears the shadow under the eye.

Hayden Panettiere

Actress and Singer

HAYDEN SAYS

"Beauty is not a fact, it's an opinion."

Like this look? I gave this same look to Nicole in "Picture Perfect" (page 137). For Hayden, I chose a deeper green shimmer eye shadow. I applied the shadow along the lower lash line and blended it higher toward Hayden's brow bone.

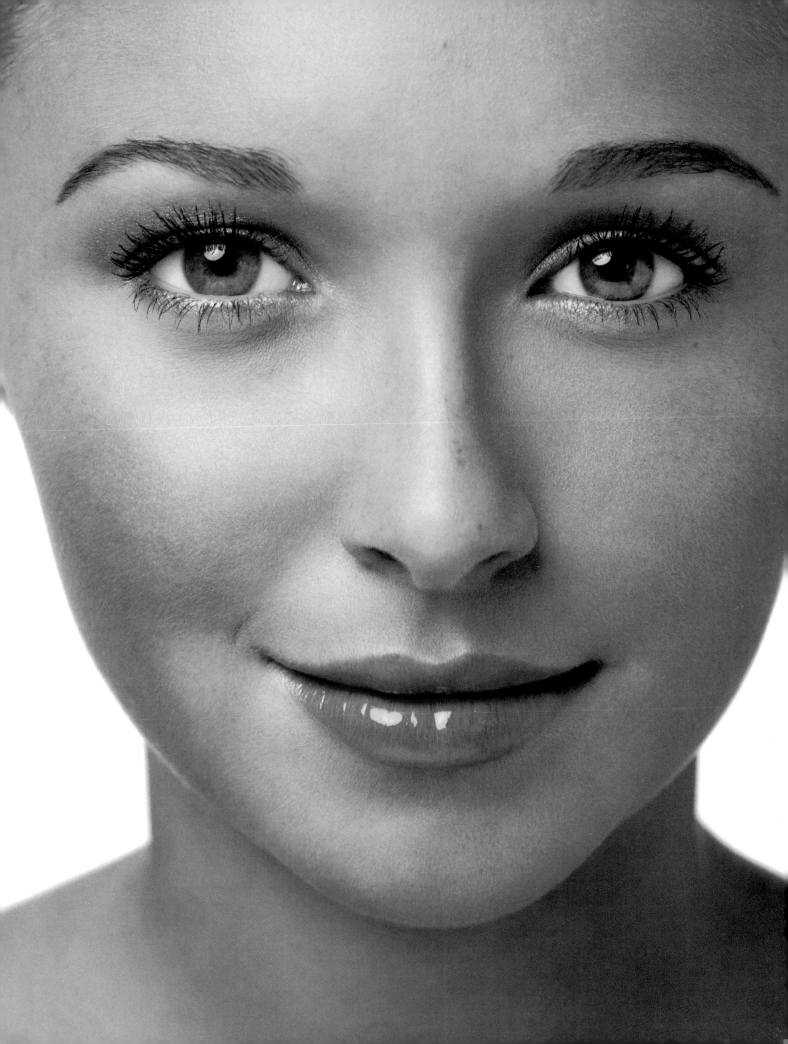

Dashenka

Dashenka is determined to carve out a space all her own. Her strong spirit is also gracious and generous, proving that ambition isn't always blind and is often beautiful.

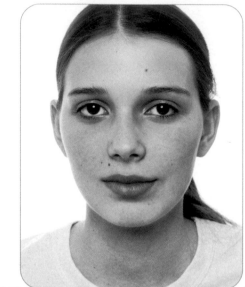

BEFORE: I covered a few spots, brightened the area under her eyes, and cleaned and shaped her eyebrows.

Tools
Toner
Tinted moisturizer with SPF
Concealer
Face/Translucent powder
Powder bronzer
Caramel lip gloss
Brow gel
Medium brown eyebrow pencil
White shimmer powder eye shadow
Lash curler
Black mascara

Truly U

The Look: Because this makeup is natural, it allows you to incorporate your own attitude into the overall look, giving it a different fla'va.

Get This Look

Step 1
Start with clean, prepped skin. Wash your face, then apply toner. Let the product soak into your skin for five minutes.

Step 2
Using clean hands, rub a tinted moisturizer with SPF on your face. Start at the center and blend out toward the ends of your face. Be sure to blend down your neck.

Step 3
Apply concealer with your *ring* fingertip, that's the one next to your pinkie. Dab in the bottom and top inner corners of your eyes and below your eyes, out and over, or wherever you see blue, gray, or red. Blend down and out by tapping the concealer into place until there are no distinct lines. Rub any leftover concealer on any redness around your nostrils and on any spots.

Step 4
Set your tinted moisturizer and concealer by lightly dusting powder over the face with a puff or a big fluffy brush.

Step 5
Wash the bronzer over the apples of your cheeks.

Step 6
Use your lip brush to apply a coat of gloss.

Step 7
Use the brush of your eyebrow gel to brush your eyebrows up and out. Fill in any gaps with the eyebrow pencil. Apply less than you think you should.

Step 8
Dust the eye shadow all over your lids and blend down into the corners of the eyes.

Step 9
Curl your lashes and apply one coat of mascara.

SCHLIPTIP: Hitting the sheets with your makeup on. Don't do it; clean that beautiful skin and let it shine spot-free in the morning!

Why It's a Winner: White eye makeup is so dramatic with richly toned skin!

What the Pros Say: "This Gurl looks beautiful, but it's her *inner peace* that shines through and shows off her face with harmonious colors and a soft glow." —Ken Pavés, celebrity hairstylist to Jessica Simpson and Eva Longoria

The Bigger Picture: You've gotta work every part of you. Be happy about all of your details. They make you who you are.

CANDY LAND

The Look: Combining a bold lip with a simple eye is just one way Dashenka looks fantastic!

SCHLIPTIP: Don't try to highlight everything in one look. Yes, you have great eyes, cheeks, and lips. But don't try to make them all pop at once. Pick eyes for one look . . . your lips for the next. Go for the cheeks on another day.

Tools
Toner
Tinted moisturizer with SPF
Concealer
Face/Translucent powder
Powder bronzer
Sheer hot pink gloss
Brow gel
Medium brown eyebrow pencil
White shimmer powder eye shadow
Lash curler
Black mascara

Get This Look

Step 1
Start with clean, prepped skin. Wash your face, then apply toner. Let the product soak into your skin for five minutes.

Step 2
Using clean hands, rub a tinted moisturizer with SPF on your face. Start at the center and blend out toward the ends of your face. Be sure to blend down your neck.

Step 3
Apply concealer with your *ring* fingertip, that's the one next to your pinkie. Dab in the bottom and top inner corners of your eyes and below your eyes, out and over, or wherever you see blue, gray, or red. Blend down and out by tapping the concealer into place until there are no distinct lines. Rub any leftover concealer on any redness around your nostrils and on any spots.

Step 4
Set your tinted moisturizer and concealer by lightly dusting powder over the face with a puff or a big fluffy brush.

Step 5
Wash bronzer over the apples of your cheeks.

Step 6
Apply the gloss with your lip brush.

Step 7
Use the brush of your eyebrow gel to brush your eyebrows up and out. Fill in any gaps with the eyebrow pencil. Apply less than you think you should.

Step 8
Dust the eye shadow all over the lids and blend down into the corner of the eyes.

Step 9
Curl your lashes and apply one coat of mascara.

Why It's a Winner: Simply changing your lips completely changes this look!

What the Pros Say: "This Gurl doesn't look like a dreamer, she looks like a believer." —Susie Crippen, designer for J Brand Jeans

The Bigger Picture: Keep your head up. Walking into a room proudly—with a big smile on your face—can make you the most interesting person in the room.

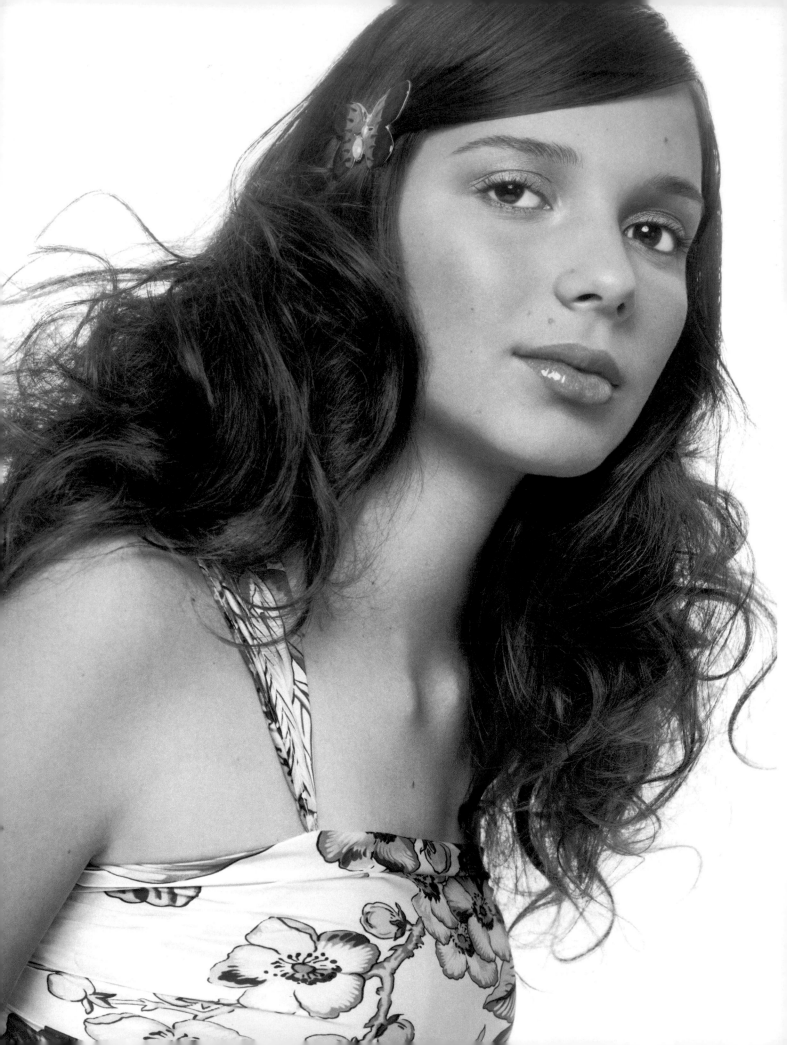

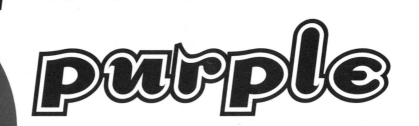

precious purple

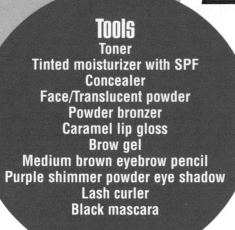

Tools
Toner
Tinted moisturizer with SPF
Concealer
Face/Translucent powder
Powder bronzer
Caramel lip gloss
Brow gel
Medium brown eyebrow pencil
Purple shimmer powder eye shadow
Lash curler
Black mascara

The Look: Even though the colors in this look are light and bright, it's perfect for an evening out.

Get This Look

Step 1
Start with clean, prepped skin. Wash your face, then apply toner. Let the product soak into your skin for five minutes.

Step 2
Using clean hands, rub a tinted moisturizer with SPF on your face. Start at the center and blend out toward the ends of your face. Be sure to blend down your neck.

Step 3
Apply concealer with your *ring* fingertip, that's the one next to your pinkie. Dab in the bottom and top inner corners of your eyes and below your eyes, out and over, or wherever you see blue, gray, or red. Blend down and out by tapping the concealer into place until there are no distinct lines. Rub any leftover concealer on any redness around your nostrils and on any spots.

Step 4
Set your tinted moisturizer and concealer by lightly dusting translucent powder over the face with a puff or a big fluffy brush.

Step 5
Wash the bronzer over the apples of your cheeks.

Step 6
A sweep of gloss applied with a lip brush leaves your mouth perfect.

Step 7
Use the brush of your eyebrow gel to brush your eyebrows up and out. Fill in any gaps with the eyebrow pencil. Apply less than you think you should.

Step 8
With an eye shadow brush, wash the eye shadow all over the lids, just to the crease. Be sure to blend the edge of the shadow to keep it soft and flattering.

Step 9
Curl your lashes and apply one coat of mascara.

Why It's a Winner: Wow! Using purple shadow instead of white really warms up this look. With a color change, Dashenka has a whole new look!

What the Pros Say: "The contrast of soft and bright colors makes Dashenka's creamy skin the focus of this look!" —Erica Westheimer, Hollywood movie producer

The Bigger Picture: This look is all about getting noticed. Your first step is giving *yourself* the attention you deserve.

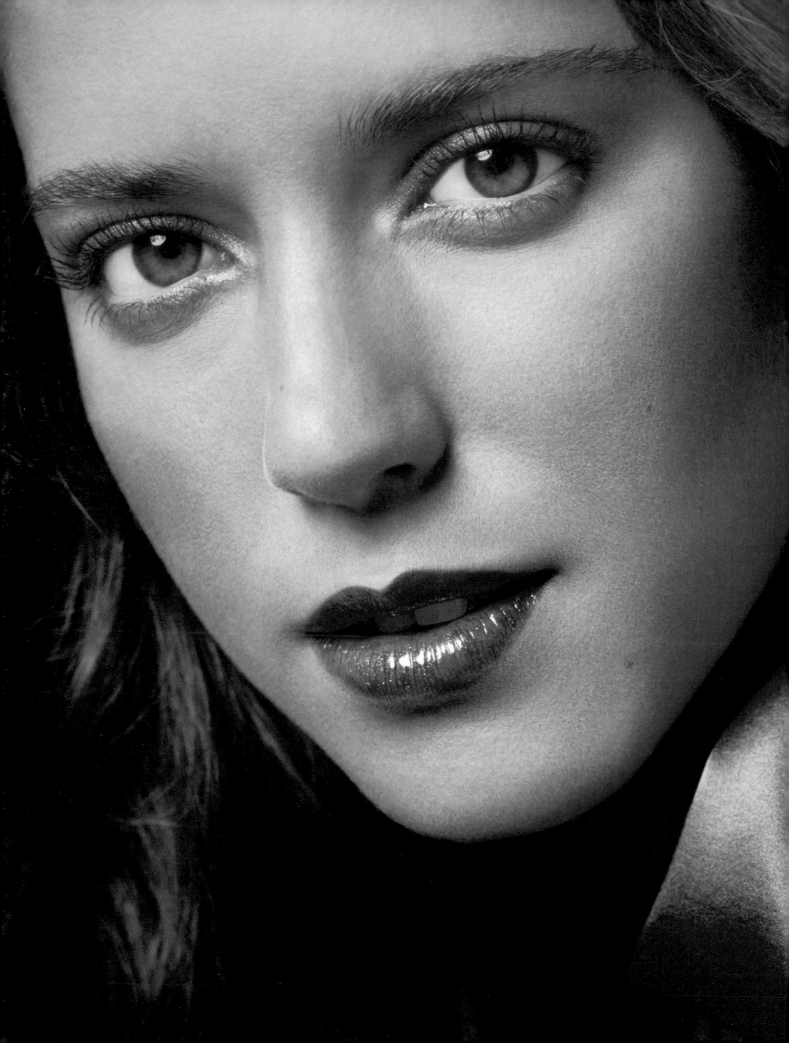

Ana Claudia Talancón

Actress

This gorgeous Gurl has worked hard to get where she is. Ana Claudia is extremely grateful for every opportunity. She gets to do the things she loves and appreciates every moment. She's the ultimate happy, compassionate, and beautiful soul.

LIKE THIS LOOK? I gave this look to Olea in "Think Pink" (page 71). Ana Claudia's look is exactly the same, except she's wearing a bronze shimmer shadow on her eyes.

attitude

There are things in life you just can't control. What you can control is how you react. And the key is having a positive attitude!

Positive thoughts become positive outcomes. It's a chain reaction.

HAPPINESS IS A CHOICE!
CHOOSE TO BE HAPPY!

dream big!

Nothing shines like a bright future. Whether you already know what you want to do in your life, or you're still trying to figure it all out, **DREAM BIG!**

Dream as big as you can imagine and then dream bigger. Your motivation to make your dream a reality will take care of the rest!

Brittany

Smart and sharp, Brittany sees potential around every corner and is among the first to hear the sound of opportunity knocking. This Glamour Gurl dreams big, aims high, and is sure to go far.

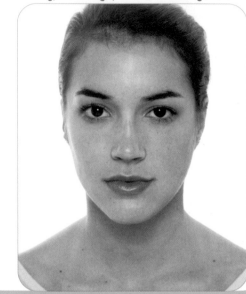

BEFORE: Brittany tends to get dark circles around her eyes, a bit of uneven skin tone, and a few spots. I fixed these and also chose to clean and shape her eyebrows.

Tools
Toner
Tinted moisturizer with SPF
Concealer
Face/Translucent powder
Caramel crème blush
Sheer beige lip gloss
Brow gel
Medium brown eyebrow pencil
Shimmery blue powder eye shadow
Lash curler
Black mascara

retro glam

The Look: Kind of funky, without being over the top. You could definitely wear this to the movies!

Get This Look

Step 1
Start with clean, prepped skin. Wash your face, then apply toner. Let the product soak into your skin for five minutes.

Step 2
Using clean hands, rub a tinted moisturizer with SPF on your face. Start at the center and blend out toward the ends of your face. Be sure to blend down your neck.

Step 3
Apply concealer with your *ring* fingertip, that's the one next to your pinkie. Dab in the bottom and top inner corners of your eyes and below your eyes, out and over, or wherever you see blue, gray, or red. Blend down and out by tapping the concealer into place until there are no distinct lines. Rub any leftover concealer on any redness around your nostrils and on any spots.

Step 4
Set your tinted moisturizer and concealer by lightly dusting powder over your face with a puff or a big fluffy brush.

Step 5
Using your fingers, apply the crème blush to the apples of the cheeks, blending out toward your ears.

Step 6
Apply your lip gloss with a brush.

Step 7
Use the brush of your eyebrow gel to brush your eyebrows up and out. Fill in any gaps with the eyebrow pencil. Apply less than you think you should.

Step 8
Wash the eye shadow lightly all over your lids and blend just to the crease.

Step 9
Curl your lashes and apply one coat of mascara.

Why It's a Winner: The steel-blue shimmery shadow makes a bold statement that brings out the eyes, without having to line them with black.

What the Pros Say: "Wow! This Gurl is just so fabulous! She's got that extra something special. She shows it off without showing off." —Tracy Bayne, fashion photographer for Beyoncé Knowles

The Bigger Picture: Brittany normally wears this scarf around her neck, but today she's using it as a fun hair accessory. Tomorrow it could be a belt. Get creative!

snow angel

The Look: Crisp, clean, and festive! Perfect for a holiday party or a Gurled-up day of snowboarding or shoppping at the mall.

Tools
Toner
Tinted moisturizer with SPF
Concealer
Face/Translucent powder
Shimmery peach crème blush
Sheer peach lip gloss
Brow gel
Medium brown eyebrow pencil
White shimmer crème eye shadow
Lash curler
Black mascara

Get This Look

Step 1
Start with clean, prepped skin. Wash your face, then apply toner. Let the product soak into your skin for five minutes.

Step 2
Using clean hands, rub a tinted moisturizer with SPF on your face. Start at the center and blend out toward the ends of your face. Be sure to blend down your neck.

Step 3
Apply concealer with your *ring* fingertip, that's the one next to your pinkie. Dab in the bottom and top inner corners of your eyes and below your eyes, out and over, or wherever you see blue, gray, or red. Blend down and out by tapping the concealer into place until there are no distinct lines. Rub any leftover concealer on any redness around your nostrils and on any spots.

Step 4
Set your tinted moisturizer and concealer by lightly dusting powder over the face with a puff or a big fluffy brush.

Step 5
Using your fingers, apply the crème blush to the apples of your cheeks.

Step 6
Coat lips with the gloss.

Step 7
Use the brush of your eyebrow gel to brush your eyebrows up and out. Fill in any gaps with the eyebrow pencil. Apply less than you think you should.

Step 8
Using your fingers, wash the eye shadow all over your lids: Fill in and blend the product from your lash line to just below your brow bone. Then, to open up the eye, apply the eye shadow in the corners of your eyes, *above* and *below* your *lower* lid.

Step 9
Curl your lashes and apply one coat of mascara.

Why It's a Winner:
Opening up the eye with a bit of white "shadow" makes a big difference!

What the Pros Say:
"I love this look. It's clean and has *the glow* without looking too frosty. Sometimes white eye shadow looks chalky and this TOTALLY doesn't."
—Solange Knowles, actress, singer, and songwriter

The Bigger Picture:
The easiest way to get this bright-eyed look is by actually *being* bright-eyed. As it turns out, sleep and good nutrition actually *do* improve the way you look!

Solange Knowles

Actress, Singer, and Songwriter

This beautiful Gurl knows great makeup! She's sharp and funny, with a quick wit. Better than anything else, she's easygoing, with the confidence of a Gurl who knows she's good at what she does.

LIKE THIS LOOK? I gave this same look to Dashenka in "Precious Purple" (page 47). For Solange I added a smudge of purple shadow to her lower lash line, and a smudge of black kohl pencil along her top lashes.

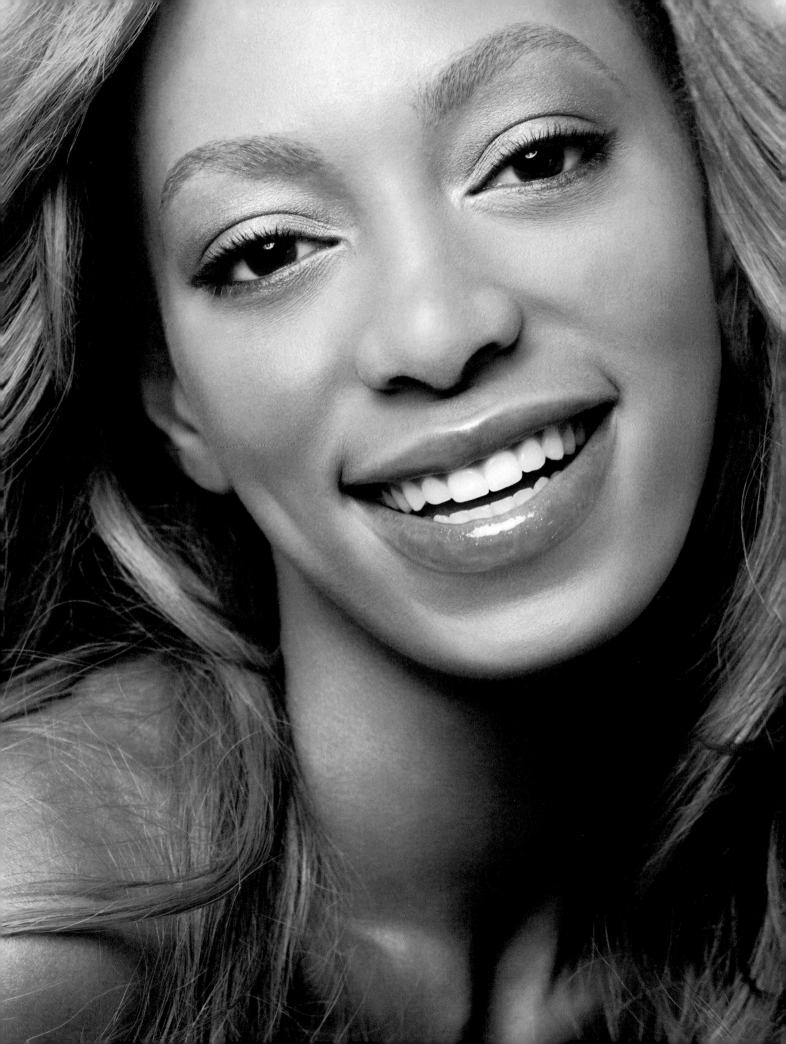

Janica

This exotic beauty has soul. She's smart and confident and knows where she's headed.

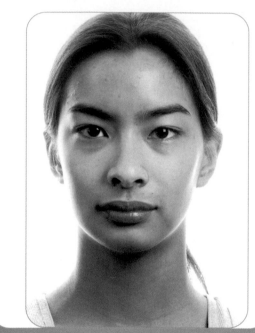

BEFORE: Janica's beauty is timeless; however, her expressive eyes do have some dark shading underneath and her skin has just a few spots. She benefits from having her complexion evened out and her brow line cleaned up.

Tools
Toner
Tinted moisturizer with SPF
Concealer
Face/Translucent powder
Bright pink pressed powder blush
Rose lip gloss
Brow gel
Medium brown eyebrow pencil
Medium brown shimmer crème eye shadow
Gold crème eyeshadow
Lash curler
Black mascara

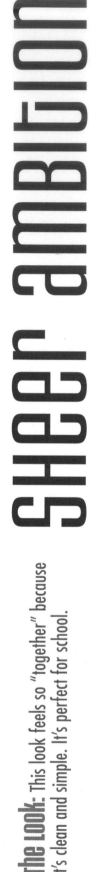

sheer ambition

The Look: This look feels so "together" because it's clean and simple. It's perfect for school.

Get This Look

Step 1
Start with clean, prepped skin. Wash your face, then apply toner. Let the product soak into your skin for five minutes.

Step 2
Using clean hands, rub a tinted moisturizer with SPF on your face. Start at the center and blend out toward the ends of your face. Be sure to blend down your neck.

Step 3
Apply concealer with your *ring* fingertip, that's the one next to your pinkie. Dab in the bottom and top inner corners of your eyes and below your eyes, out and over, or wherever you see blue, gray, or red. Blend down and out by tapping the concealer into place until there are no distinct lines. Rub any leftover concealer on any redness around your nostrils and on any spots.

Step 4
Set your concealer by lightly tapping translucent powder over it with a puff or a fluffy brush.

Step 5
Using a blush brush, apply the blush to the apples of your cheeks, keeping the edges soft and blended.

Step 6
Use a lip brush to apply the gloss over your lips.

Step 7
Use the brush of your eyebrow gel to brush your eyebrows up and out. Fill in any gaps with the eyebrow pencil. Apply less than you think you should.

Step 8
Apply a thin swipe of the brown shimmer crème eye shadow next to the lash line. Then, above that, blend in the gold-colored crème eye shadow to the crease and the rest of the way to your brow line.

Step 9
Curl lashes and apply one coat of mascara to the *top* lashes only.

Why It's a Winner: Gurl confidence conveys a sense of success—the best kind of pretty!

What the Pros Say: "This Gurl breaks all the beauty stereotypes of Asian, African-American, Latina, and Caucasian Gurlz. You can't place her ethnicity, and that makes her unique and exotic; she embodies the wild new beauty frontier! She could work as a model every day." —James Charles, Director of New Faces, L.A. Models agency

The Bigger Picture: Looking *under*done is a great way to look together.

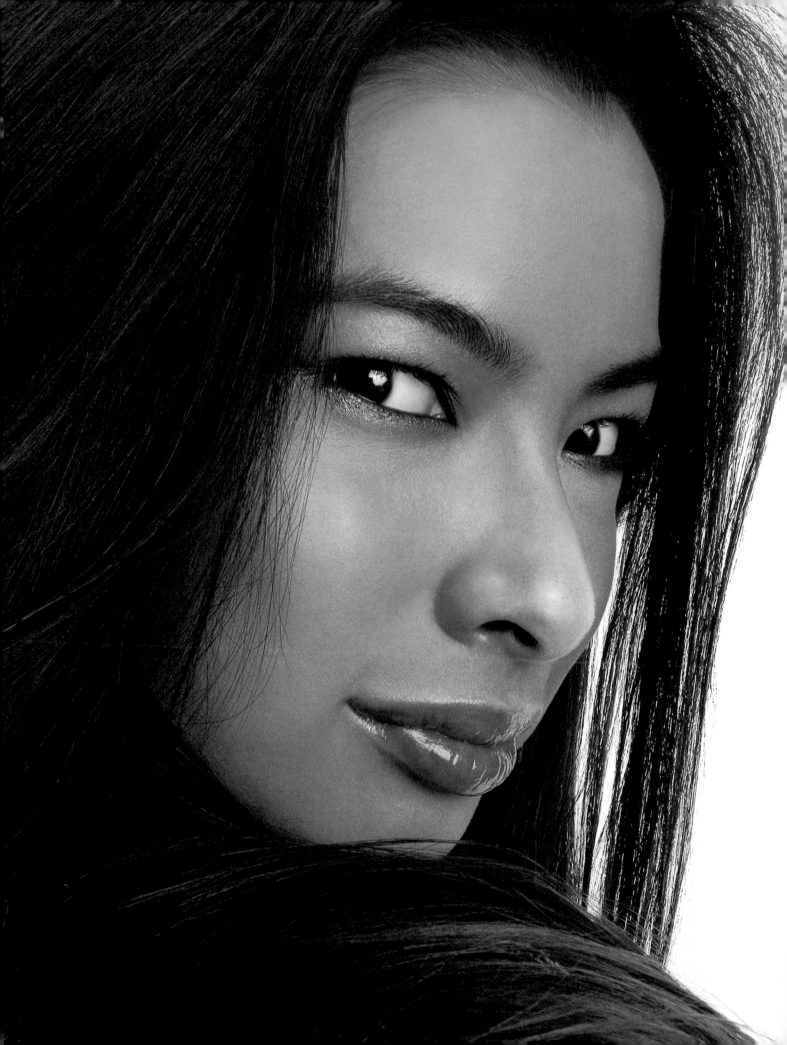

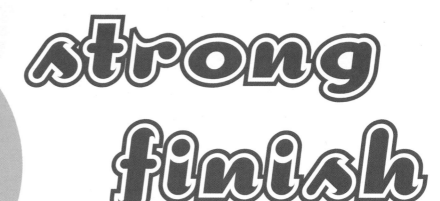

Tools
Toner
Tinted moisturizer with SPF
Concealer
Face/Translucent powder
Peach pressed powder blush
Rose-tinted lip balm
Brow gel
Medium brown eyebrow pencil
Black kohl eyeliner pencil
Sheer camel crème eye shadow
Sparkly gunmetal-gray kohl pencil
Cotton swab
Lash curler
Black mascara

The Look: Go from daytime party to nighttime drama by highlighting eyes with a smoky finish!

Get This Look

Step 1
Start with clean, prepped skin. Wash your face, then apply toner. Let the products soak into your skin for five minutes.

Step 2
Using clean hands, rub a tinted moisturizer with SPF on your face. Start at the center and blend out toward the ends of your face. Be sure to blend down your neck.

Step 3
Apply concealer with your *ring* fingertip, that's the one next to your pinkie. Dab in the bottom and top inner corners of your eyes and below your eyes, out and over, or wherever you see blue, gray, or red. Blend down and out by tapping the concealer into place until there are no distinct lines. Rub any leftover concealer on any redness around your nostrils and on any spots.

Step 4
Set your concealer by lightly tapping translucent powder over it with a puff or a fluffy brush.

Step 5
Using a brush, apply the blush to the apples of your cheeks, keeping the edges soft and blended.

Step 6
Use a lip brush to apply the lip balm.

Step 7
Use the brush of your eyebrow gel to brush your eyebrows up and out. Fill in any gaps with the eyebrow pencil. Apply less than you think you should.

Step 8
Now for your eyes. First, line the bottom *inner* rim of each eye with the soft black kohl pencil. Then, apply the eye shadow to the top lid, up to the brow. Blend well. To finish off the look with the sparkly gunmetal-gray kohl pencil, line your lower lid and smudge the line with a cotton swab.

Step 9
Curl lashes and apply one coat of mascara to the *top* lashes only.

Why It's a Winner: This look is mysterious and modern!

What the Pros Say: "This Gurl has a plan!"
—Andrew Matusik, photographer for Hilary Duff

The Bigger Picture: Bringing out eyes also brings out the drama, but notice how everything else in this look is subtle? *That's* the secret to looking glam.

Sophia Bush

Actress

Sophia is the kind of Gurl who will put you at ease right away. She's honest and super-kind. She has a great sense of style and it shows. She's so beautiful she can walk into a room with no makeup on and still have all eyes on her.

LIKE THIS LOOK? I gave this same look to Piper in "Glam Rock" (page 179). For Sophia, I swapped out Piper's gray shimmer eye shadow for an amethyst shimmer eye shadow applied with the same technique. Instead of clear gloss, I chose a camel crème gloss for Sophia.

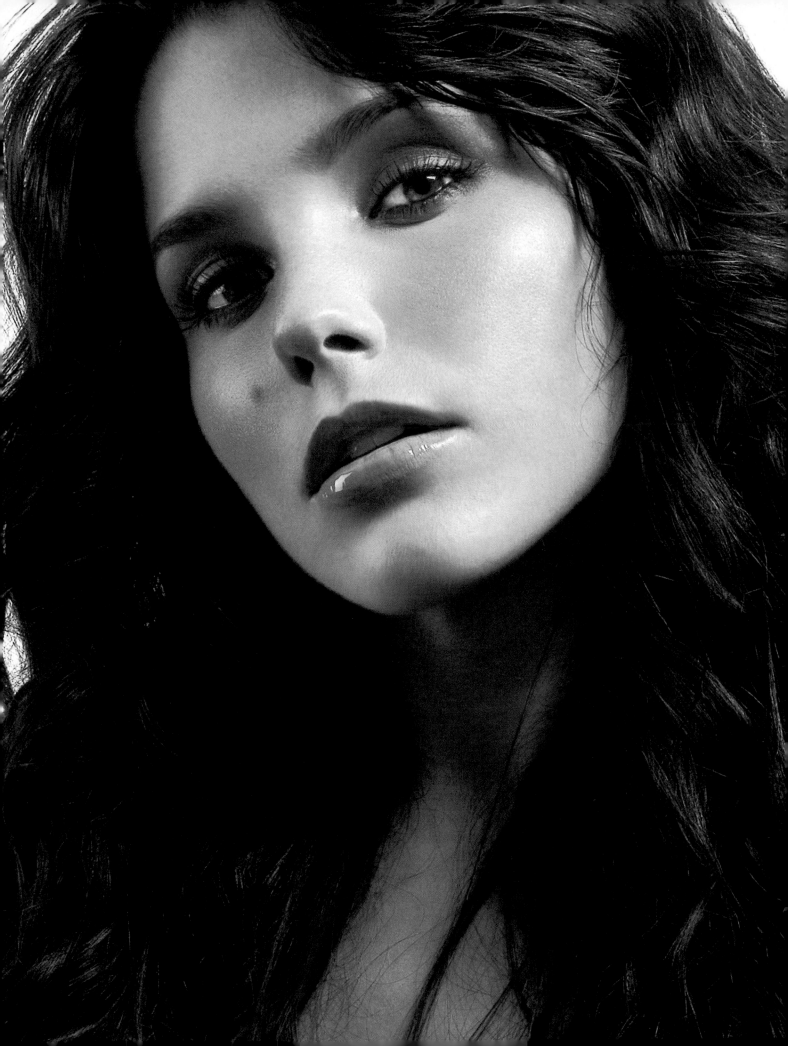

find your voice

Ever claimed to love a certain song, when you've never actually heard it? Or told all your friends you hated a movie, when you hadn't seen it? Feeling like you have to agree with others is a powerful urge. Fight it.

Understand why you feel the way you do. Form your own opinions.

You don't have to defend who you are. Don't dishonor yourself just to please others. Learn to trust yourself. Believing in yourself is the best way to become a leader and break from the crowd.

Real Smartz come in many different flavors:

Book Smartz: doing great in school!

Street Smartz: common sense to make sure everyone at the party gets home safely!

Emotional Smartz: giving great advice to your friends!

Social Smartz: being able to talk to anybody!

How many of these smartz do you have? Make a point of working on all your smartz, not just those rewarded by grades in school. Many times the best answers in life come when you put all of your smartz together.

smartz

Olea

Olea is a crazy contradiction: a Gurl who loves motocross as much as she loves makeup. If ever you think that being a fierce tomboy stops you from being a beautiful, sophisticated Gurl, think of Olea and think *again*.

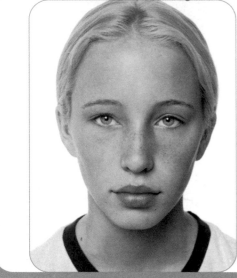

BEFORE: I tamed Olea's tomboy brows, brightened the area underneath her eyes, and covered a few spots and some redness around her nose.

Tools
Toner
Moisturizer with SPF
Concealer
Face/Translucent powder
Light peach powder blush
Caramel lip gloss
Brow gel
Blonde eyebrow pencil
Lash curler
Black mascara

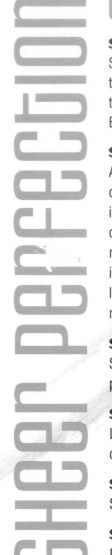

Sheer Perfection

Get This Look

Step 1
Start with clean, prepped skin. Wash your face, then apply toner and a light moisturizer with SPF. Let the products soak into your skin for five minutes. Blot away any excess with a tissue.

Step 2
Apply concealer with your *ring* fingertip, that's the one next to your pinkie. Dab in the bottom and top inner corners of your eyes and below your eyes, out and over, or wherever you see blue, gray, or red. Blend down and out by tapping the concealer into place until there are no distinct lines. Rub any leftover concealer on any redness around your nostrils and on any spots.

Step 3
Set your concealer by lightly tapping translucent powder over it with a puff or a fluffy brush.

Step 4
Lightly dust the blush on the apples of your cheeks and blend out toward the ears.

Step 5
Sweep the lip gloss over your lips.

Step 6
Use the brush of your eyebrow gel to brush your eyebrows up and out. Fill in any gaps with the eyebrow pencil. Apply less than you think you should.

Step 7
Curl your lashes and apply one coat of mascara.

Why It's a Winner: This is the perfect example of how natural makeup can be mesmerizing.

What the Pros Say: "The makeup here is so light you can see how beautiful this Gurl really is." —Shinko Iura, celebrity wardrobe stylist to Claire Danes and Taryn Manning

The Bigger Picture: This look is all about keeping it *simple*. Do you ever feel that rolling with the crowd *complicates* your life? Don't be afraid to get away from the crew and focus on your own priorities every once in a while.

the look: This natural look is perfect for anything you do during the day.

mellow yellow

The Look: This sunny look is perfect for a weekend day *or* an evening out.

Tools
Toner
Moisturizer with SPF
Concealer
Translucent powder
Caramel-colored crème blush
Brow gel
Blonde eyebrow pencil
Yellow powder eye shadow
Lash curler
Black mascara

Get This Look

Step 1
Start with clean, prepped skin. Wash your face, then apply toner and a light moisturizer with SPF. Let the products soak into your skin for five minutes. Blot away any excess with a tissue.

Step 2
Apply concealer with your *ring* fingertip, that's the one next to your pinkie. Dab in the bottom and top inner corners of your eyes and below your eyes, out and over, or wherever you see blue, gray, or red. Blend down and out by tapping the concealer into place until there are no distinct lines. Rub any leftover concealer on any redness around your nostrils and on any spots.

Step 3
Set your concealer by lightly tapping translucent powder over it with a puff or a fluffy brush.

Step 4
Using your fingers, apply the blush on the apples of your cheeks.

Step 5
Take a lip brush and swipe the blush on your *lips* as well!

Step 6
Use the brush of your eyebrow gel to brush your eyebrows up and out. Fill in any gaps with the eyebrow pencil. Apply less than you think you should.

Step 7
Using an eye shadow brush, dust yellow powder eye shadow from the lash line to the brow bone, keeping the edges soft and blended.

Step 8
Curl your lashes and apply one coat of mascara.

SCHLIPTIP ON MASCARA: Many Gurlz make the mistake of "pumping" the mascara wand into the tube in order to get more product out. Don't do it. Pumping the wand only pushes in air that will dry out your mascara and promote the growth of bacteria. Instead, *twirl* your mascara wand, by rubbing the wand against the sides of the tube, to get additional product on your wand.

Why It's a Winner: This yellow is a fresh alternative to the typical neutral shadows.

What the Pros Say: "This look reminds me of the fashion runways, but it's so wearable and pretty. I almost can't believe it's so bold." —Jenny Cho, celebrity hairstylist to Ashlee Simpson and Michelle Trachtenberg

The Bigger Picture: The yellow in this look is hot. But notice, no overall skin coverage. Not every look calls for tinted moisturizer. Cherish your opportunities to be *real*.

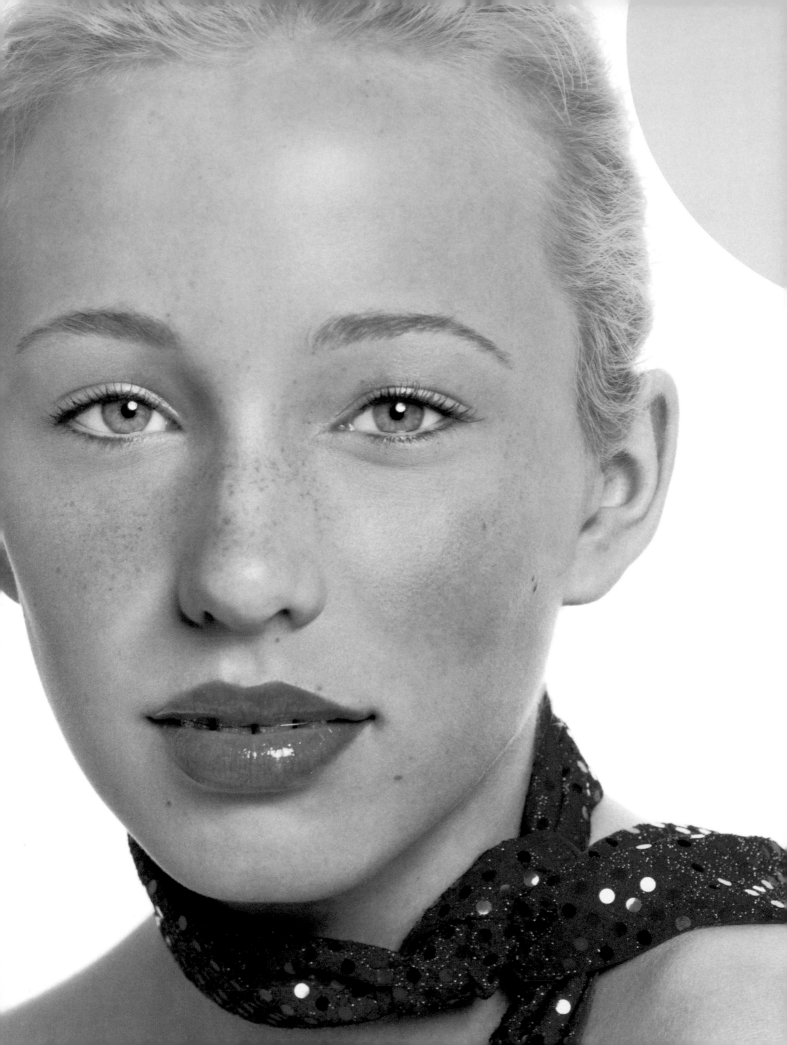

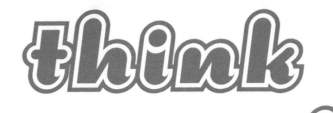

think pink

Tools
Toner
Moisturizer with SPF
Concealer
Face/Translucent powder
Pink powder blush
Hot pink lip gloss
Brow gel
Blonde eyebrow pencil
Gold powder eye shadow
Lash curler
Black mascara

The Look: Sassy! This look takes pink to the next level. Perfect for a day or evening out with your friends or your favorite guy.

Get This Look

Step 1
Start with clean, prepped skin. Wash your face, then apply toner and a light moisturizer with SPF. Let the products soak into your skin for five minutes. Blot away any excess with a tissue.

Step 2
Apply concealer with your *ring* fingertip, that's the one next to your pinkie. Dab in the bottom and top inner corners of your eyes and below your eyes, out and over, or wherever you see blue, gray, or red. Blend down and out by tapping the concealer into place until there are no distinct lines. Rub any leftover concealer on any redness around your nostrils and on any spots.

Step 3
Set your concealer by lightly tapping translucent powder over it with a puff or a fluffy brush.

Step 4
Lightly dust the blush on the apples of the cheeks and blend out toward your ears.

Step 5
With a lip brush, apply your gloss.

Step 6
Use the brush of your eyebrow gel to brush your eyebrows up and out. Fill in any gaps with the eyebrow pencil. Apply less than you think you should.

Step 7
Using an eye shadow brush, dust your eye shadow from the lash line to the brow bone, softening the color as you move up.

Step 8
Curl your lashes and apply one coat of mascara.

Why It's a Winner:
Perfectly polished, this look keeps eyes and cheeks soft, and creates impact with a bright pink lip.

What the Pros Say:
"This Gurl can wear her makeup any way she wants because she knows she looks great. She gives a feeling of a very outgoing, simple style that doesn't need tons of makeup to define her." —Robert Steinken, celebrity hairstylist to Sandra Bullock

The Bigger Picture:
This look features a better version of pink. What actions will make *you* a *better* version of *you*?

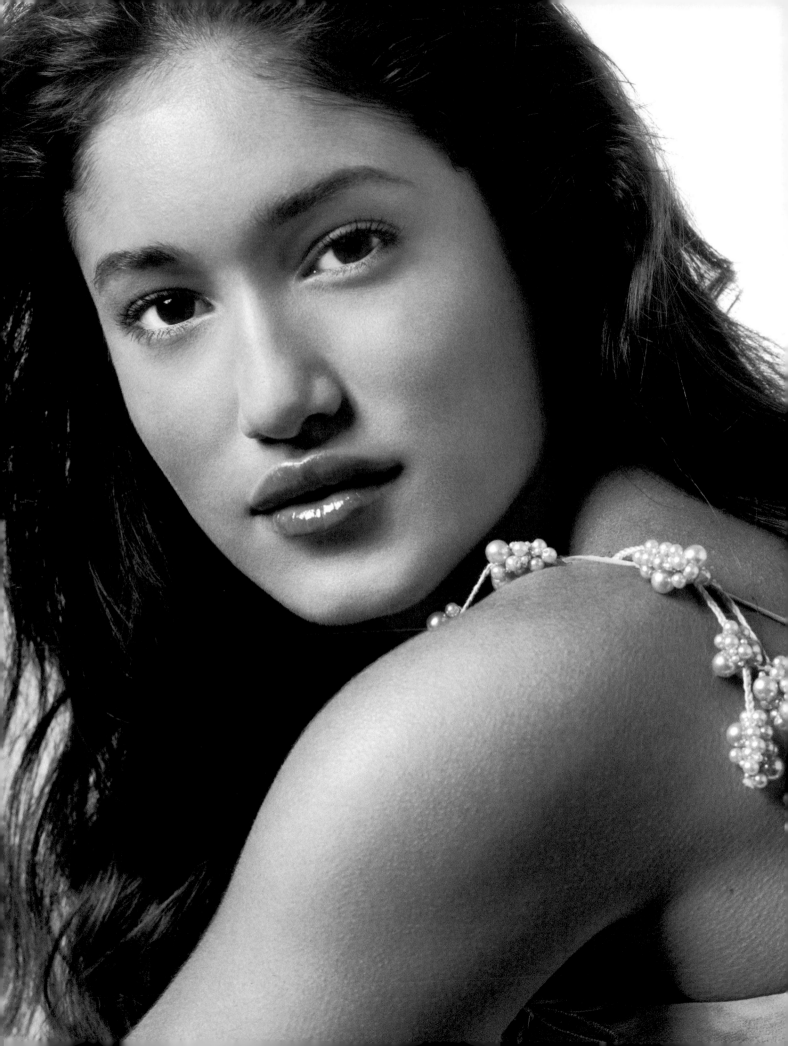

Q'Orianka Kilcher

Actress, Singer, and Songwriter

When I think of gorgeous Q'Orianka, I immediately think of the word *proud*. She's proud of her family heritage and the journey that brought her where she is now. She has an extraordinary story that includes her first job as a street performer. She's beautiful in every way, because she's so down-to-earth. Regardless of how high her star rises, she will never forget her roots.

Like This Look? I gave this same look to Amanda in "All Dolled Up" (page 24). See how Q'Orianka gets the "natural look" with a gold crème eye shadow? The color is a bit different, but the technique is the same!

Q'Orianka Kilcher

Actress, Singer, and Songwriter

Never dumb yourself down to try to fit in. There is nothing prettier than an intelligent Gurl. Smart is beautiful!

Like this look? I gave this same look to Jinsol in "Isle of Style" (page 127). Q'Orianka adapted it by smudging a little bit of the gold shadow along her lower lash line. Everything else is the same in Jinsol's look! Isn't it interesting how the same technique can look so different on different Glamour Gurlz?

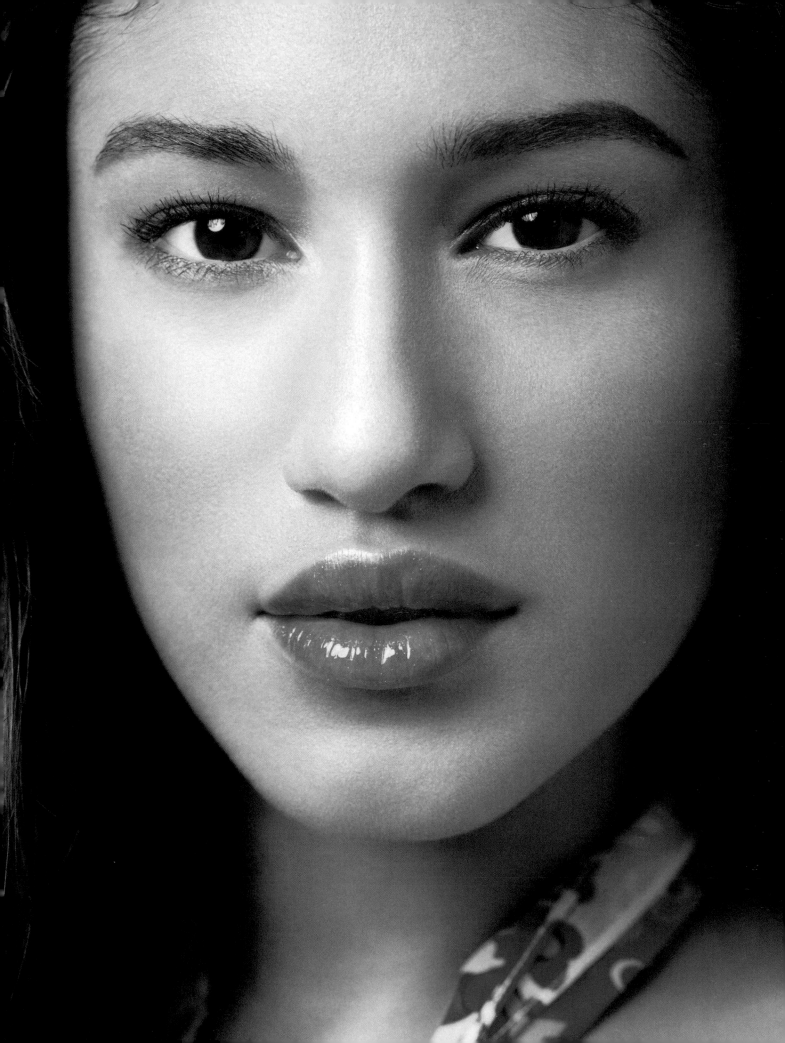

global gurl

Take an interest in what's going on in the rest of the world. Technology has made the globe a much smaller place, connecting you to people all over this world as if they lived next door. Why not use technology to learn about other places and other Gurlz' experiences? Before you know it, you'll have friends in South Africa, Italy, Sweden, or Brazil. The more you learn about what's out there and how other Gurlz are living, the more global you'll become!

everyday extraordinary

One of the best ways to have an extraordinary day is to volunteer to help others. You'll get out of your head and into someone else's reality, and you'll be amazed by how much of a difference you can make in another person's life!

Beauty Skooled:
Francis, Kimberly, and Franchesca

like this look? Monica has the same one in "Up Front" (page 120). I used the exact same makeup on all the Gurlz! I love the way each Gurl made the look her own by honoring it with her individual beauty and style.

Jennifer Freeman

Actress

Jennifer's an extraordinary beauty who's tapped into what's really important: what's on the inside. Her attitude is: If it's not broken, don't fix it. Work with what you've got!

LIKE THIS LOOK? It's the same look as Lena in "Downtown Princess" (page 89). Instead of flat brown eye shadow I used a cocoa brown shimmer shadow and blended it up to the brow bone. A sheer pink lip gloss and peach crème blush on the cheeks complete the look.

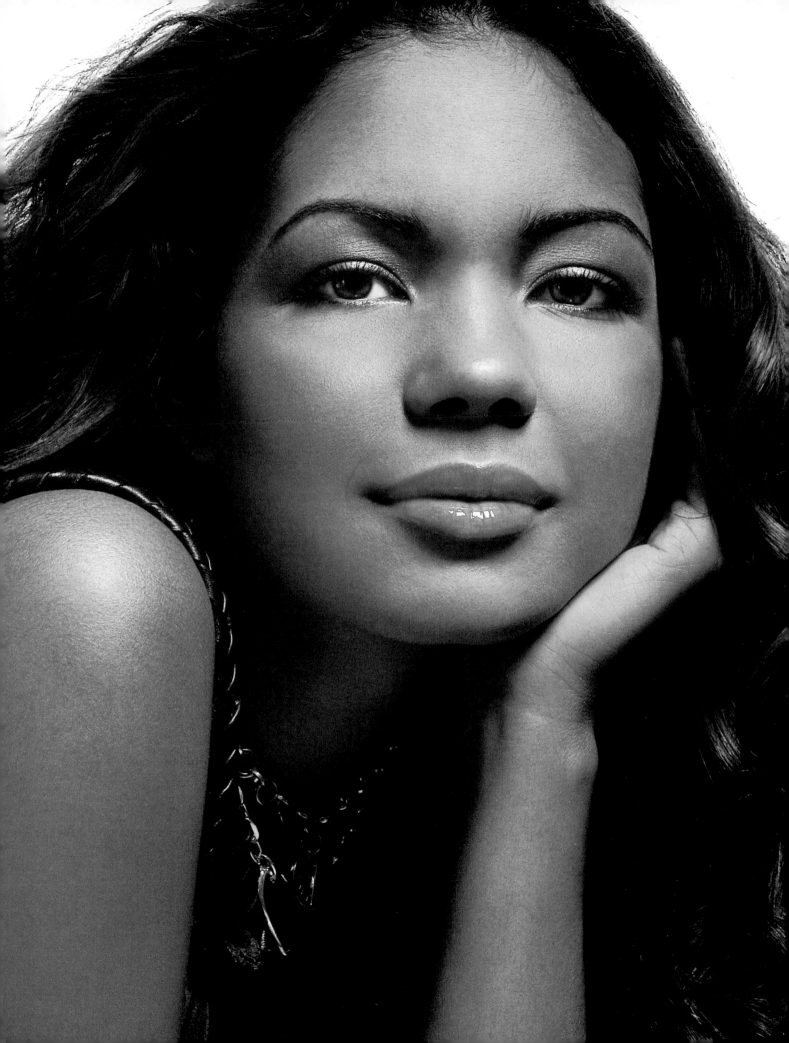

own it!

Ever spot a trendsetter and wonder: How does she pull that off? How do some people make taking risks look so effortless? Gurl, it's all about owning it!

No one can wear your look like you can, so put some confidence in those steps, be your magnificent self, and fill up that spotlight with your style.

confidence

It takes a confident girl to give a compliment to a pretty girl she sees, but it also takes confidence to accept a compliment.

What do you do when some-one tells you that you look beautiful? Do you shrug it off, or do you smile and say, "Thank you"? There is noth-ing wrong with recognizing that you are pretty.

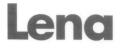

Lena

Still waters run deep with Lena. This beautiful Gurl doesn't demand the spotlight, but *boy* does she shine when it's on her. Lena reminds me that the softest voices often have the most important things to say.

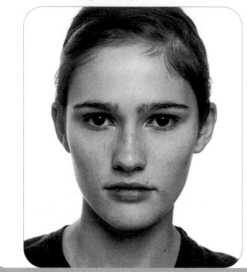

BEFORE: I tamed her spirited brows by shaping and cleaning, brightened the area under her eyes, and covered a few spots and some redness around her nose.

Tools
Toner
Tinted moisturizer with SPF
Concealer
Face/Translucent powder
Peach crème blush
Natural lip liner pencil in a shade just slightly darker than your natural lip tone
Peach lip gloss
Brow gel
Light brown eyebrow pencil
Bronze shimmer crème eye shadow
Lash curler
Black mascara

sweetheart

the look: A great look for school, the mall, the movies, or dinner with your friends *or your parents.*

Get This Look

Step 1
Start with clean, prepped skin. Wash your face, then apply toner. Let the products soak into your skin for five minutes.

Step 2
Using clean hands, rub a tinted moisturizer with SPF on your face. Start at the center and blend out toward the ends of the face. Be sure to blend down your neck.

Step 3
Apply concealer with your *ring* fingertip, that's the one next to your pinkie. Dab in the bottom and top inner corners of your eyes and below your eyes, out and over, or wherever you see blue, gray, or red. Blend down and out by tapping the concealer into place until there are no distinct lines. Rub any leftover concealer on any redness around your nostrils and on any spots.

Step 4
Set your tinted moisturizer and concealer by lightly dusting powder over your face with a puff or a big fluffy brush.

Step 5
Using your fingers, apply the crème blush on the apples of your cheeks, keeping the edges soft and blended.

Step 6
Softly line along your natural lip line with the lip liner.

Step 7
Apply the gloss with your lip brush. Blend the gloss and lip liner together.

Step 8
Use the brush of your eyebrow gel to brush your eyebrows up and out. Fill in any gaps with the eyebrow pencil. Apply less than you think you should.

Step 9
Use your finger to wash the eye shadow all over your lids and blend up toward the brow bone.

Step 10
Curl your lashes and apply one coat of mascara.

Why It's a Winner: It's super sheer and gives you all the glamour you need!

What the Pros Say: "This look is girly and sweet, without looking too young or too simple. Love it!"—Ken Pavés, celebrity hairstylist to Jessica Simpson and Eva Longoria

The Bigger Picture: Makeup *simplified* . . . you're out the door in five minutes or less with this polished look. That leaves you plenty of free time for all the other things you'd rather do!

angel face

The Look: This look is so fresh and clean, you could wear it to the mall, to dinner with your Gurlz, *and* to math class.

Tools
Toner
Tinted moisturizer with SPF
Concealer
Face/Translucent powder
Pink crème blush
Natural lip liner pencil in a shade just slightly darker than your natural lip tone
Shiny pink lip gloss
Brow gel
Light brown eyebrow pencil
Gold shimmer crème eye shadow
Lash curler
Black mascara

Get This Look

Step 1

Start with clean, prepped skin. Wash your face, then apply toner. Let the product soak into your skin for five minutes.

Step 2

Using clean hands, rub a tinted moisturizer with SPF on your face. Start at the center and blend out toward the ends of the face. Be sure to blend down your neck.

Step 3

Apply concealer with your *ring* fingertip, that's the one next to your pinkie. Dab in the bottom and top inner corners of your eyes and below your eyes, out and over, or wherever you see blue, gray, or red. Blend down and out by tapping the concealer into place until there are no distinct lines. Rub any leftover concealer on any redness around your nostrils and on any spots.

Step 4

Set your tinted moisturizer and concealer by lightly dusting powder over your face with a puff or a big fluffy brush.

Step 5

Using your fingers, apply the blush to the apples of your cheeks, keeping the edges soft and blended.

Step 6

Softly line along your natural lip line with the lip liner.

Step 7

Apply lip gloss with your brush. Blend the gloss and lip liner together.

Step 8

Use the brush of your eyebrow gel to brush your eyebrows up and out. Fill in any gaps with the eyebrow pencil. Apply less than you think you should.

Step 9

Wash the eye shadow all over your lids and blend up toward the brow bone.

Step 10

Curl your lashes and apply one coat of mascara.

Why It's a Winner: The warm pink blush and gloss really flatter Lena's skin tone.

What the Pros Say: "I love how happy she looks in this picture. What's prettier than a beautiful smile?" —Susie Crippen, fashion designer for J Brand Jeans

The Bigger Picture: Trust your instincts. Even if a color combination doesn't work on other Gurlz, you never know—you could be the Gurl for whom it looks great!

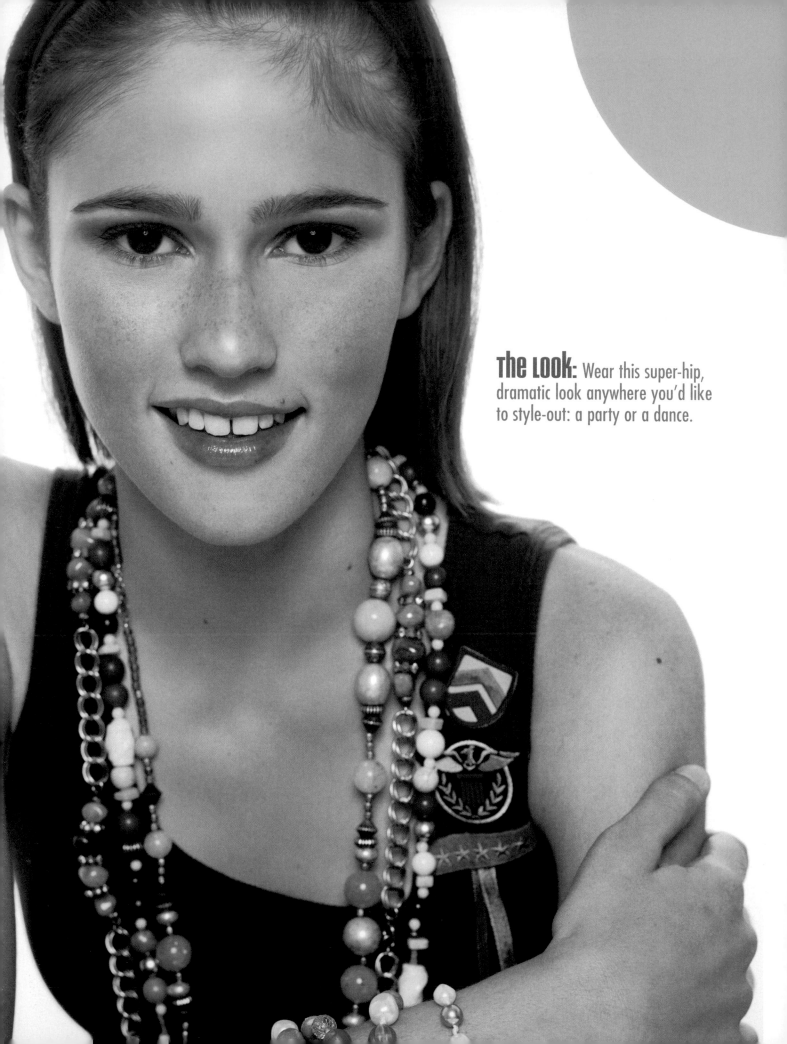

the LOOK: Wear this super-hip, dramatic look anywhere you'd like to style-out: a party or a dance.

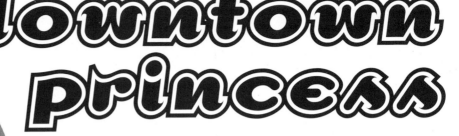

downtown princess

Tools
Toner
Tinted moisturizer with SPF
Concealer
Face/Translucent powder
Peach crème blush
Natural lip liner pencil in a shade just
slightly darker than your natural lip tone
Shiny pink lip gloss
Brow gel
Light brown eyebrow pencil
Medium brown pressed eye shadow
Lash curler
Black mascara

Get This Look

Step 1
Start with clean, prepped skin. Wash your face, then apply toner. Let the product soak into your skin for five minutes.

Step 2
Using clean hands, rub a tinted moisturizer with SPF on your face. Start at the center and blend out toward the ends of the face. Be sure to blend down your neck.

Step 3
Apply concealer with your *ring* fingertip, that's the one next to your pinkie. Dab in the bottom and top inner corners of your eyes and below your eyes, out and over, or wherever you see blue, gray, or red. Blend down and out by tapping the concealer into place until there are no distinct lines. Rub any leftover concealer on any redness around your nostrils and on any spots.

Step 4
Set your tinted moisturizer and concealer by lightly dusting powder over your face with a puff or a big fluffy brush.

Step 5
Using your fingers, apply the blush to the apples of your cheeks, keeping the edges soft and blended.

Step 6
Softly line along your natural lip line with the lip liner.

Step 7
Apply your lip gloss with a brush. Blend the gloss and lip liner together.

Step 8
Use the brush of your eyebrow gel to brush your eyebrows up and out. Fill in any gaps with the eyebrow pencil. Apply less than you think you should.

Step 9
Using your brush, wash the eye shadow all over your lids and blend up toward the brow bone.

Step 10
Curl your lashes and apply one coat of mascara.

Why It's a Winner: This look has edge, without being overdone.

What the Pros Say: "This Gurl knows what she's all about. She seems sure of herself. There's strength in those eyes." —Enzo Angileri, celebrity hairstylist to Charlize Theron

The Bigger Picture: This look changes one single item—the powder eye shadow—and suddenly the perception is darker, completely different. If brown eye shadow can do this, imagine how piercings, tattoos, and other alterations affect the way you are perceived. Think before you ink, Gurl.

The Veronicas

Singers and Songwriters

The Veronicas are super-cute. Jess and Lisa complement each other, not only with their talent, but also with their confidence and self-esteem. They have a great sense of style and make a statement wherever they go. They're kind and generous to each other. You can tell there is a genuine respect and love between these twin sisters.

like this look? I gave this same look to Margarita in "Urban Edge" (page 156). The Veronicas' eyes are lined the same way as Margarita's. The twins' look is different because before I applied the liner, I added a sand shimmery crème eye shadow from the lash line to the brow and then smudged the liner up into the crease with a shimmery cocoa brown pressed powder eye shadow. I also smudged and blended the lower lash line with a light touch of the cocoa brown eye shadow and replaced Margarita's pink blush and lip gloss with apricot-colored ones.

Caitlin

Not only is she beautiful, she's got a heart of gold. This Gurl spends little time worrying about her own style and more time focusing on others. She regularly volunteers in her community and in other places around the world!

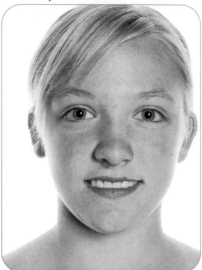

BEFORE: I brightened up under Caitlin's eyes and shaped her brows.

Tools
Toner
Tinted moisturizer with SPF
Concealer
Face/Translucent powder
Peach pressed powder blush
Sheer pink lip gloss
Brow gel
Blonde eyebrow pencil
Shimmery gold powder eye shadow
Lash curler
Black mascara

prom princess

The Look: This natural look still seems dressed up enough for going out.

Get This Look

Step 1
Start with clean, prepped skin. Wash your face, then apply toner. Let the product soak into your skin for five minutes.

Step 2
Apply tinted moisturizer with SPF the same color as your skin to even out skin tone.

Step 3
Apply concealer with your *ring* fingertip, that's the one next to your pinkie. Dab in the bottom and top inner corners of your eyes and below your eyes, out and over, or wherever you see blue, gray, or red. Blend down and out by tapping the concealer into place until there are no distinct lines. Rub any leftover concealer on any redness around your nostrils and on any spots.

Step 4
Set your concealer by lightly tapping translucent powder over it with a puff or a fluffy brush.

Step 5
Using a blush brush, apply the blush to the apples of your cheeks, keeping the edges soft and blended.

Step 6
Sweep the gloss over your lips.

Step 7
Use the brush of your eyebrow gel to brush your eyebrows up and out. Fill in any gaps with the eyebrow pencil. Apply less than you think you should.

Step 8
Dip your eye shadow brush into the eye shadow and blend it onto your lids, starting at the lash line and working up to the crease.

Step 9
Curl your lashes and apply one coat of mascara, only on the *top* lashes.

Why It's a Winner: Gold shimmer really brings out the warm tones in Caitlin's coloring.

What the Pros Say: "I think Caitlin is a natural beauty whose self-confidence shines through with an amazing glow. . . . Radiant!" —Jessica Simpson, actress, singer, and songwriter

The Bigger Picture: Sure, sometimes you see bronzer applied for "glow." But a *true* radiant glow is something you just can't fake. So glow, Gurl, *glow*.

SHOW Stopper

The Look: The little splash of color here makes the eyes *pop!* and adds definition.

Get This Look

Step 1
Start with clean, prepped skin. Wash your face, then apply toner. Let the product soak into your skin for five minutes.

Step 2
Apply tinted moisturizer with SPF the same color as your skin to even out skin tone.

Step 3
Apply concealer with your *ring* fingertip, that's the one next to your pinkie. Dab in the bottom and top inner corners of your eyes and below your eyes, out and over, or wherever you see blue, gray, or red. Blend down and out by tapping the concealer into place until there are no distinct lines. Rub any leftover concealer on any redness around your nostrils and on any spots.

Step 4
Set your concealer by lightly tapping translucent powder over it with a puff or a fluffy brush.

Step 5
Skip the blush for this look; we're going to emphasize the *eyes.*

Step 6
Cover your lips with a clear gloss for a natural glow.

Step 7
Use the brush of your eyebrow gel to brush your eyebrows up and out. Fill in any gaps with the eyebrow pencil. Apply less than you think you should.

Step 8
Blend the eye shadow onto your lids, starting at the lash line and working up to your crease.

Step 9
Dip an eyeliner brush into the same eye shadow and brush on just *below* your *lower* lash line for subtle emphasis.

Step 10
Curl your lashes and apply one coat of mascara to top lashes only.

Why It's a Winner:

Balancing color on the eye with a blushless cheek is what pulls this whole look together.

What the Pros Say:

"Could she be any prettier? Her eyes look so happy. You can just see that she's a great Gurl." —Joanna

The Bigger Picture:

Just as you carefully make choices about which accessories to add to your look, balance out your makeup choices so that it's *you*—and not your makeup or your clothing—that stands out.

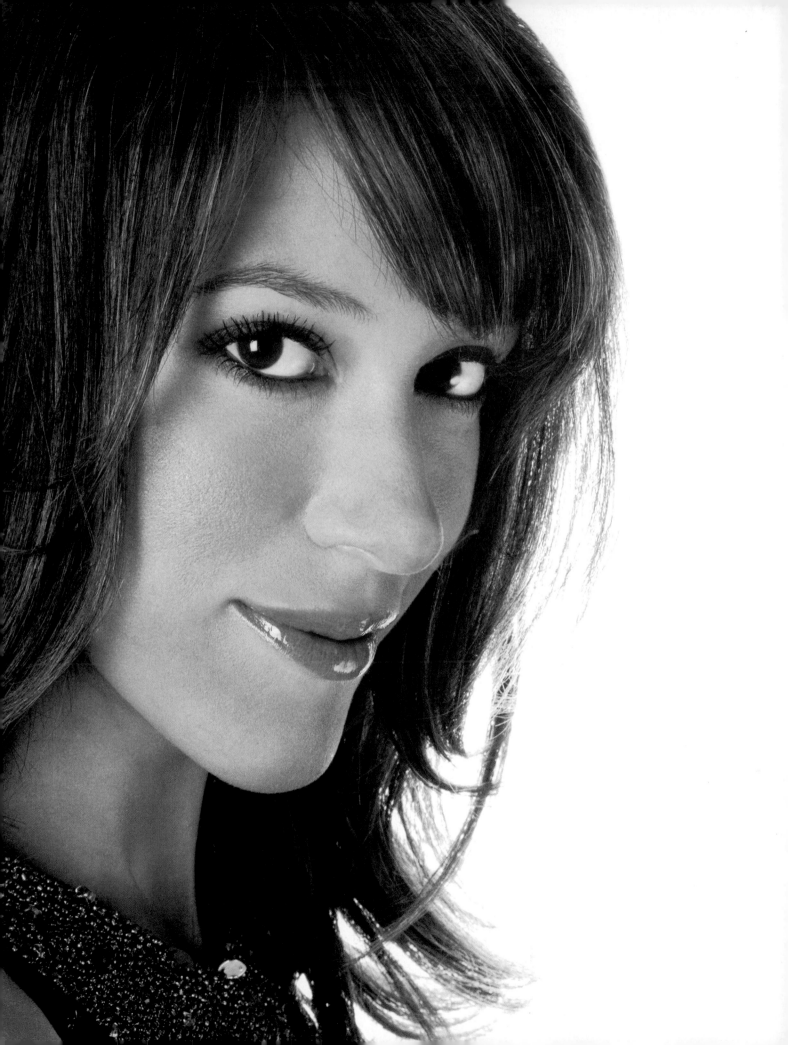

Haylie Duff

Actress, Singer, and Songwriter

As I sat in front of this gorgeous Gurl I realized: Behind those beautiful eyes are a powerful mind and a generous heart. This Glamour Gurl is all about helping and inspiring others!

HAYLIE SAYS:

"Real glamour and beauty is not just mascara, Chanel N°5 perfume, and perfect lip gloss, it's being a role model, being beautiful on the inside, and caring more about others than you do about yourself."

Like This Look?

I gave this same look to Jessica in "City Pretty" (page 146). I brightened up the look for Haylie by switching the outside liner and pressed powder eye shadow from Jessica's black to a rich copper for Haylie.

focus forward

You will get what you think you deserve. If you believe you deserve a great life, a great life—and everything it has to offer—is what you will have.

clownin'!

Have fun with life. Smile, play, and laugh. Laugh loud and laugh a lot. Nothing is prettier than a happy Gurl.

Respect yourself and others will follow.

ginger snap

Ali

Super sweet and truly genuine, Ali loves her freckles, as she should; they are beautiful kisses from the sun!

BEFORE: Ali's freckles give her that something special. I chose to brighten up dark circles under her eyes and cover a few spots *without* covering her freckles—I love them!

The Look: Drama for redheads who don't want tons of color to overwhelm the naturally dramatic color palette of their complexion.

Tools
Toner
Tinted moisturizer with SPF
Concealer
Face/Translucent powder
Peach powder blush
Clear lip gloss
Brow gel
Light brown eyebrow pencil
Dark copper powder eye shadow
White eyeliner pencil
Lash curler
Black mascara

Get This Look

Step 1
Start with clean, prepped skin. Wash your face, then apply toner. Let the product soak into your skin for five minutes.

Step 2
Using clean hands, apply a tinted moisturizer on your face. Start at the center and blend out toward the ends of the face. Be sure to blend down your neck.

Step 3
Apply concealer with your *ring* fingertip, that's the one next to your pinkie. Dab in the bottom and top inner corners of your eyes and below your eyes, out and over, or wherever you see blue, gray, or red. Blend down and out by tapping the concealer into place until there are no distinct lines. Rub any leftover concealer on any redness around your nostrils and on any spots.

Step 4
Set your tinted moisturizer with SPF and concealer by lightly dusting powder over the face with a puff or a big fluffy brush.

Step 5
Lightly dust the blush on the apples of your cheeks.

Step 6
Using a brush, apply clear gloss to your lips.

Step 7
Use the brush of your eyebrow gel to brush your eyebrows up and out. Fill in any gaps with the eyebrow pencil. Apply less than you think you should.

Step 8
Wash the eye shadow all over, from the lash line to the brow bone. Blend out the edges.

Step 9
Now for the fun part. Take a *white* eyeliner pencil and line the *inside* of your bottom lid, to open up your eyes.

Step 10
Curl your lashes and apply one coat of mascara.

Why It's a Winner: Using *white* eyeliner on the inside of the eye completely changes the shape of the eye. In some cases it can make the eye look bigger.

What the Pros Say: "Ali told me that she's always been super-self-conscious about being so tall. Can you believe it? But that's the way it is: Petite Gurlz wish they were taller and taller Gurlz wish they were smaller! Crazy, right?" —Joanna

The Bigger Picture: Remember that we are all different. That's a good thing! Can you imagine how boring it would be if we all looked exactly alike? Every Glamour Gurl has her own individual beauty.

SCHLIPTIP: Notice how tinted moisturizer just evens out your complexion, without covering your freckles? Looks great!

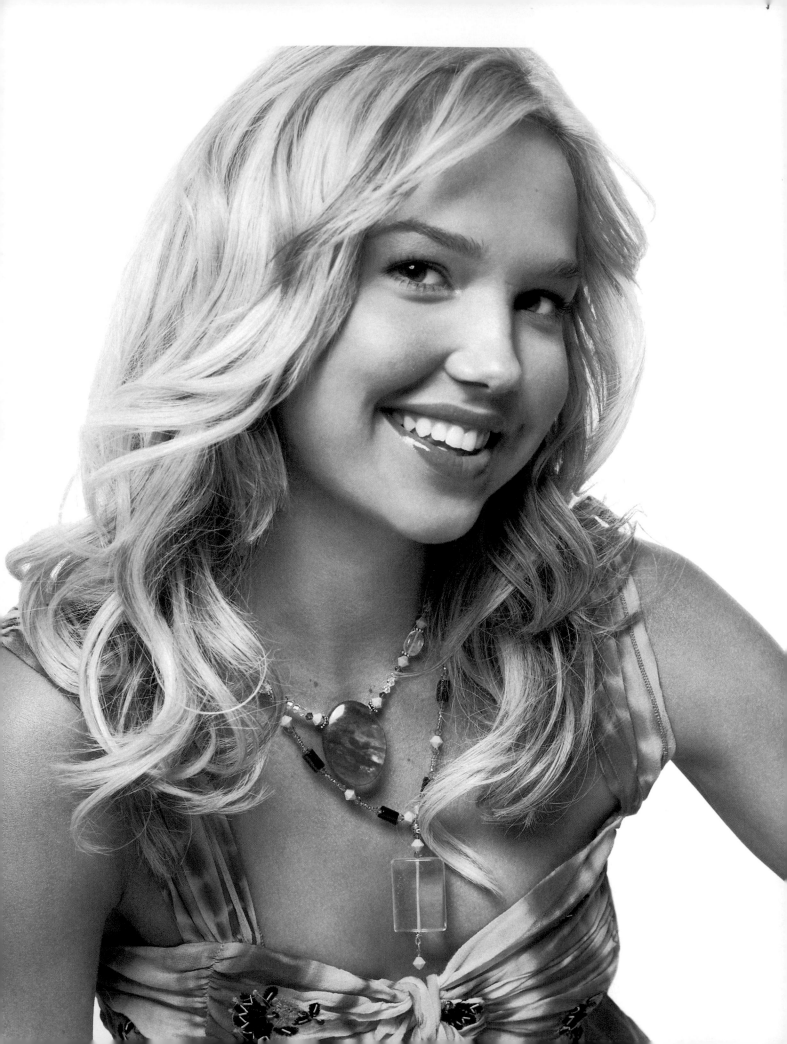

Arielle Kebbel

Actress

Arielle is such a gorgeous Gurl with a heart of gold! When she described what it felt like to see her scars erased in photographs that were supposed to be of her, I could completely relate to the experience of learning to love yourself—scars and all. Arielle is an amazing beauty inside and out!

ARIELLE SAYS

"When I first started doing photo shoots, I discovered they would digitally remove my scars. But the face I saw wasn't mine. So now I insist they use the real me . . . scars and all."

Like This Look? I gave this same look to Christine in "Urban Cowgurl" (page 106). For Arielle, I warmed up her eyes with a gold shimmer crème eye shadow. Her cheek is the same as Christine's, but she pairs her eyes with a tangerine shimmer lip gloss.

play big!

How do you become a winner in the game of life? Everyone is dealt a certain hand: You may have a good hand or the worst one ever. The important thing is not what you're dealt, but how you play the game.

Get out there and get in the game! And when you do, don't play small! Give it your all and make your mark!

It is not what you have but how you *use* what you have!

step to it!

Everybody has goals. From getting into college to growing out your hair, the same strategy applies. It's the little steps that will take you the distance. So whether you plan to reach your goal in a week, a month, or a year, realize that everyday actions and small changes make really big things happen.

Christine

So beautiful on the inside, Christine can't help but be beautiful on the outside. Generous, community-minded, and eager to make a difference in the world, Christine's star gets brighter every day.

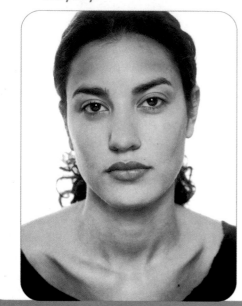

BEFORE: Christine had a few stray eyebrow hairs that needed plucking and a bit of darkness underneath the eyes.

Tools
Toner
Moisturizer with SPF
Concealer
Face/Translucent powder
Peach crème blush
Caramel lip gloss
Brow gel
Medium brown eyebrow pencil
White shimmer crème eye shadow
Lash curler
Black mascara

URBAN COWGURL

the Look: The colors are soft and pretty, yet the white shadow really makes a statement. It looks so clean!

Get This Look

Step 1
Start with clean, prepped skin. Wash your face, then apply toner and a light moisturizer with SPF. Let the products soak into your skin for five minutes. Blot away any excess with a tissue.

Step 2
Apply concealer with your *ring* fingertip, that's the one next to your pinkie. Dab in the bottom and top inner corners of your eyes and below your eyes, out and over, or wherever you see blue, gray, or red. Blend down and out by tapping the concealer into place until there are no distinct lines. Rub any leftover concealer on any redness around your nostrils and on any spots.

Step 3
Set your concealer by lightly tapping translucent powder over it with a puff or a fluffy brush.

Step 4
Using your fingers, apply the blush across your cheekbones, blending out toward your ears.

Step 5
Sweep on your lip gloss.

Step 6
Use the brush of your eyebrow gel to brush your eyebrows up and out. Fill in any gaps with the eyebrow pencil. Apply less than you think you should.

Step 7
Using the wand of your crème eye shadow, dab it all over your eyelid and blend with your fingertip up toward the brow bone.

Step 8
Curl your lashes and apply one coat of mascara.

Why It's a Winner: White shimmer shadow looks soft but still stands out!

What the Pros Say: "I always wanted to have different colored eyes, like blue or green. I tried colored contacts but they didn't look right. I came to realize how beautiful brown eyes are." —Mallory Low, actress, singer, and songwriter

The Bigger Picture: What do you like about yourself? What do you think other Gurlz like about you? You may not realize it, but some of the things you wish you could change might be on the wish list of one of your Gurlfriends!

BOHO, BaBY!

THE LOOK: The warm autumn tones are stunning on her skin.

Get This Look

Step 1
Start with clean, prepped skin. Wash your face, then apply toner and a light moisturizer with SPF. Let the products soak into your skin for five minutes. Blot away any excess with a tissue.

Step 2
Apply concealer with your *ring* fingertip, that's the one next to your pinkie. Dab in the bottom and top inner corners of your eyes and below your eyes, out and over, or wherever you see blue, gray, or red. Blend down and out by tapping the concealer into place until there are no distinct lines. Rub any leftover concealer on any redness around your nostrils and on any spots.

Step 3
Set your concealer by lightly tapping translucent powder over it with a puff or a fluffy brush.

Step 4
Lightly dust the blush across your cheekbones, blending out toward your ears.

Step 5
Using a lip brush, apply your lip gloss.

Step 6
Use the brush of your eyebrow gel to brush your eyebrows up and out. Fill in any gaps with the eyebrow pencil. Apply less than you think you should.

Step 7
Use your eye shadow brush to dip into the eye shadow and wash it all over your eyelid.

Step 8
Curl your lashes and apply one coat of mascara.

SCHLIPTIP ON KOHL: Does your best Gurlfriend want to use your kohl liner? Don't do it! Sharing eye makeup is the fastest way to get *conjunctivitis,* or "pink eye," a common eye infection that causes your eye to become red and swollen. If you must share liner, sharpen your friend's pencil a full turn before doing it and then clean the sharpener with alcohol.

Why It's a Winner: You

don't see dark orange makeup very
often, but it totally complements
Christine's coloring.

What the Pros Say:

"That's gorgeous makeup. It draws
you in to her natural beauty!"
—Q'Orianka Kilcher, actress, singer,
and songwriter

The Bigger Picture:

Makeup is *not* about being trendy,
but about looking *great*. If everyone's wearing dark orange, but your
coloring is too light to pull it off,
skip it.

THE LOOK: Liner never looked so pretty. The lime green is a refreshing change from the usual black or brown.

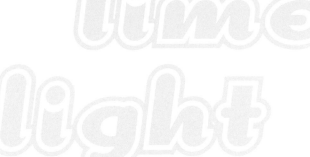

Tools
Toner
Moisturizer with SPF
Concealer
Translucent powder
Pale peach shimmer powder blush
Shiny peach lip gloss
Brow gel
Medium brown eyebrow pencil
Lime green eyeliner
Lash curler

Get This Look

Step 1
Start with clean, prepped skin. Wash your face, then apply toner and a light moisturizer with SPF. Let the products soak into your skin for five minutes. Blot away any excess with a tissue.

Step 2
Apply concealer with your *ring* fingertip, that's the one next to your pinkie. Dab in the bottom and top inner corners of your eyes and below your eyes, out and over, or wherever you see blue, gray, or red. Blend down and out by tapping the concealer into place until there are no distinct lines. Rub any leftover concealer on any redness around your nostrils and on any spots.

Step 3
Set your concealer by lightly tapping translucent powder over it with a puff or a fluffy brush.

Step 4
Lightly dust the blush across your cheekbones, blending out toward your ears.

Step 5
Using a lip brush, apply your lip gloss.

Step 6
Use the brush of your eyebrow gel to brush your eyebrows up and out. Fill in any gaps with the eyebrow pencil. Apply less than you think you should.

Step 7
Line all the way around the eye with lime green eyeliner—next to the top and bottom lashes. Keep the look bright and bold by *not* blending the line.

Step 8
Curl your lashes and you're finished.

Why It's a Winner: This look makes a strong eye, without mascara!

What the Pros Say: "I love this color combination, lips and eyebrows super-natural with a colorful, strong eye." —Hayden Panettiere, actress, singer, and songwriter

The Bigger Picture: You're an original, and your makeup should be, too. Don't be afraid to change up the color to get a fresh look going.

grace, gurl

Whether it's on the runway or in the hallway, not every look is going to be a smash.

Bottom line? Part of being a trendsetter is accepting what flops and what flies with style, grace, and a sense of humor. If your look bombs, give yourself props for having the confidence to try something new!

you have it!

Want to get that new look? You might not need to buy new makeup. You can probably create almost any new look with the products you already have in your makeup kit.

Not sure if you can pull off that new look? Close your eyes and know that you can. Tell yourself that you are pretty and that you get prettier every day. Don't believe it? Look in the mirror the next time you finish gym class. See that healthy glow? That's you!

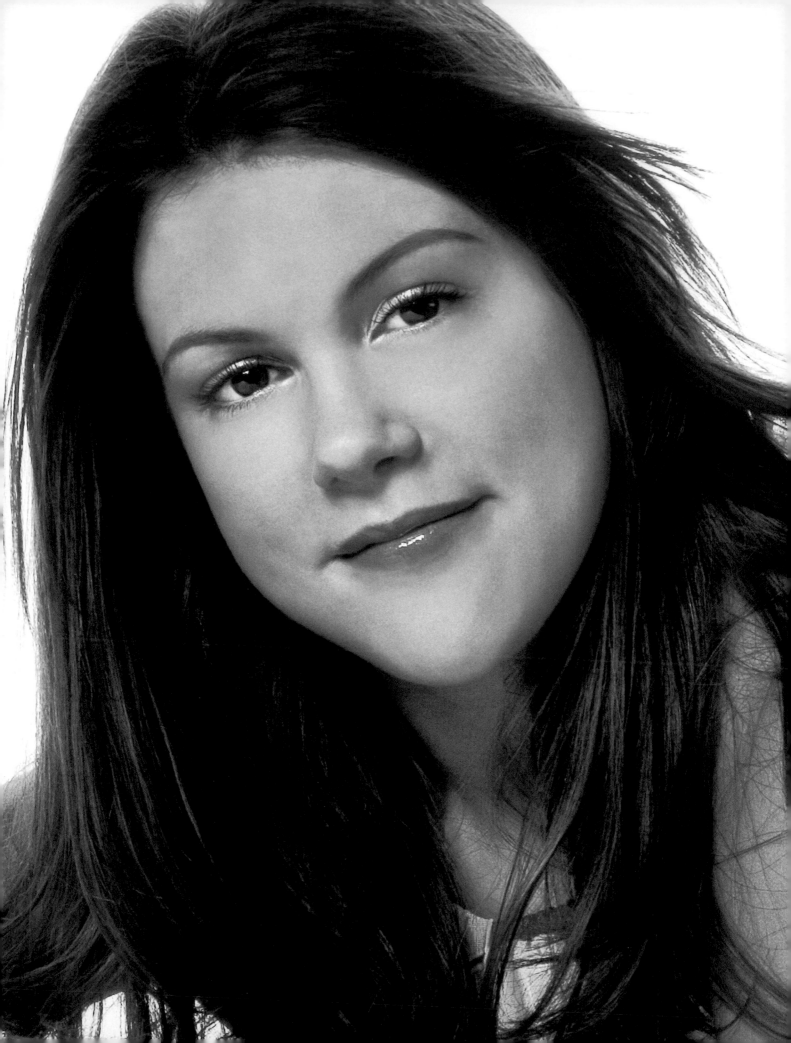

Lindsey Shaw

Actress

Adorable Lindsey is drawn to a higher beauty——the things that make a difference in this world. Her strong spirit is gracious and generous, and her ambition makes her look all the more beautiful.

Like this look? I gave this same look to Mia in "Quick Silver" (page 160). Lindsey added an ice-blue pressed powder shimmer eye shadow, layered and blended up to the brow. A sheer peach lip gloss completes her version of this look.

Sometimes hangin' solo can feel lonely or embarrassing. You might think you look out of place or like a loser, but nothing could be farther from the truth.

did'ya know

Standing alone allows you to focus your energy on yourself, not on all the other girls you're hanging with. It's like taking time to get to know *you*.

And when you have a good relationship with yourself, you will have all that you need to rise to every occasion.

Glamour Gurlz, we are *all* worthy of feeling beautiful just as we are, in our own skin. If you know this—really know it—this strong sense of self will make you look beautiful to everyone you come in contact with, every day. Look in the mirror every day and say out loud:

"I'm beautiful, you're beautiful, we are all beautiful in our skin!"
—Jessica Simpson, actress, singer, and songwriter

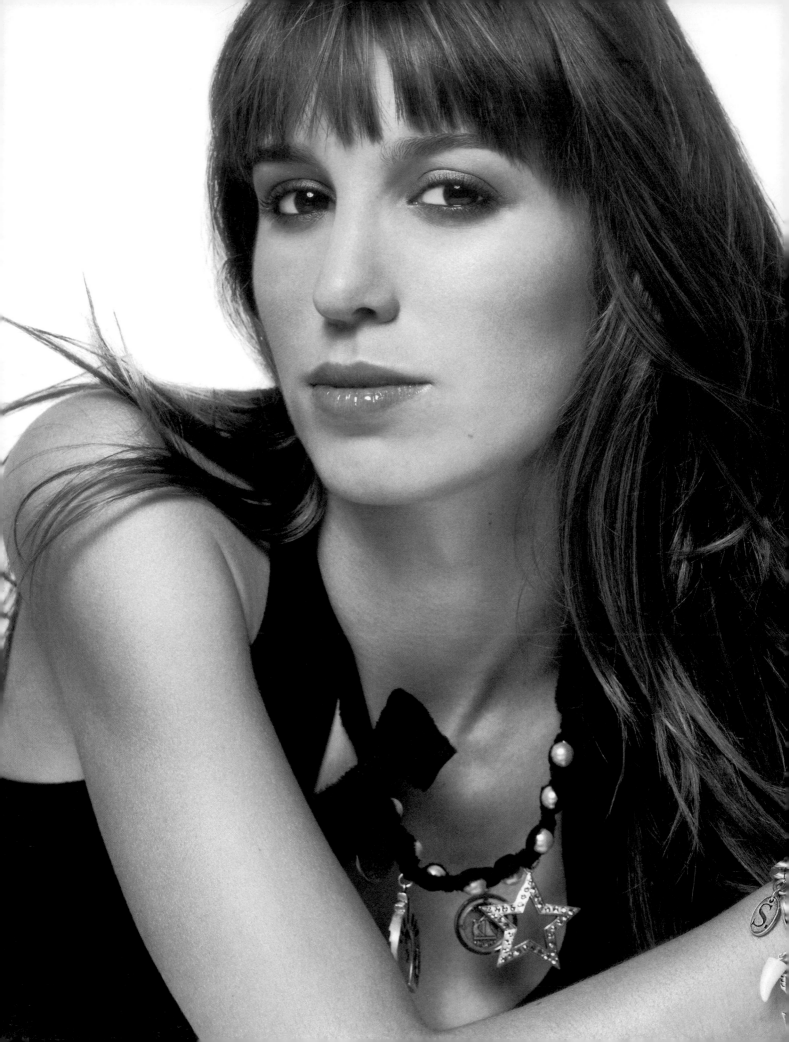

Christy Carlson Romano
Actress, Singer, and Songwriter

As I'm working on the beautiful Christy Carlson Romano—a Gurl so accomplished at such a young age—I ask her how she did it. She said to me, "I just try to take one step at a time . . . I just make sure I keep walking." Christy is a solid beauty inside and out.

LIKE THIS LOOK? I gave this same look to Janica in "Strong Finish" (page 61). Christy started with these same elements, but took it a little farther when I lined her top lash line with black kohl pencil and blended in a gunmetal shimmer pressed powder eye shadow over her lid, up to the crease. A soft coral gloss highlights her lips.

Monica

This ambitious go-getter is a social butterfly. She loves makeup and loves to experiment with new looks.

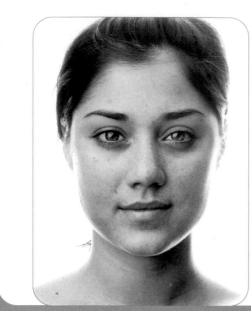

BEFORE: I chose to clean up Monica's brows, brighten dark circles under her eyes, and smooth out uneven skin tone caused by this Beach Gurl's sun exposure.

Tools
Toner
Tinted moisturizer with SPF
Concealer
Face/Translucent powder
Pale pink shimmer powder blush
Clear lip gloss
Brow gel
Medium brown eyebrow pencil
Peach powder eye shadow
Lash curler
Black mascara

Up Front

The Look: The perfect look for school or anytime you want to look finished, but as if you didn't try too hard.

Get This Look

Step 1
Start with clean, prepped skin. Wash your face, then apply toner. Let the product soak into your skin for five minutes.

Step 2
Apply tinted moisturizer with SPF, the same tone as your skin, to even out skin tone.

Step 3
Apply concealer with your *ring* fingertip, that's the one next to your pinkie. Dab in the bottom and top inner corners of your eyes and below your eyes, out and over, or wherever you see blue, gray, or red. Blend down and out by tapping the concealer into place until there are no distinct lines. Rub any leftover concealer on any redness around your nostrils and on any spots.

Step 4
Set your concealer by lightly tapping translucent powder over it with a puff or a fluffy brush.

Step 5
Using your blush brush, dust the blush on the apples of your cheeks, keeping the edges soft and blended.

Step 6
Sweep the clear gloss over your lips.

Step 7
Use the brush of your eyebrow gel to brush your eyebrows up and out. Fill in any gaps with the eyebrow pencil. Apply less than you think you should.

Step 8
Apply the eye shadow on your lids, starting at the lash line and working up to your eyebrow. Use a light, windshield-wiper motion for optimum blending.

Step 9
Curl your lashes and apply one coat of mascara to the top lashes only.

SCHLIPTIP: Bronze up. Love the beach look? Skip the sun and use bronzer instead of a crème blush for a more modern, less heavy look—especially in warm weather!

Why It's a Winner: Peach looks fantastic with richer complexions!

What the Pros Say: "This Gurl is beautiful because she has confidence from within. She wears the look from the inside out. There's confidence in her style. She owns it." —Carlos Ortiz, celebrity hairstylist to Mandy Moore and Jennifer Love Hewitt

The Bigger Picture: The healthy glow Gurlz get from being in the sun can be "applied" more safely and more quickly with a great self-tanning formula and shiny bronzer. Try it before you bake!

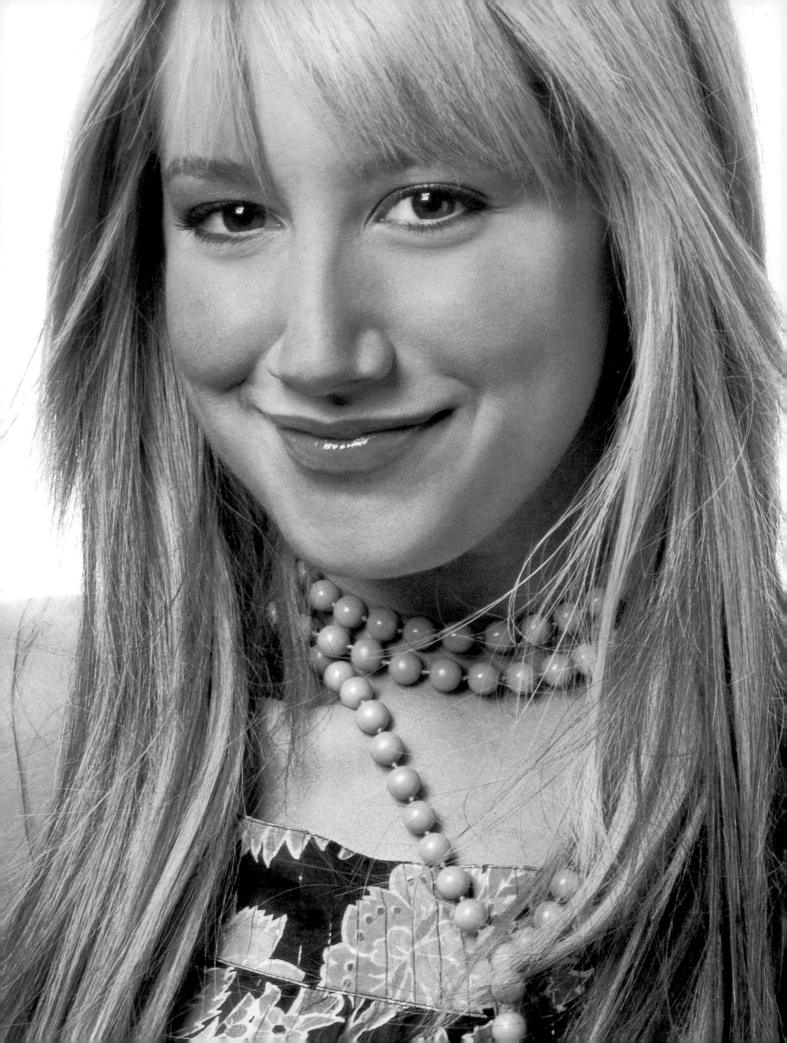

Ashley Tisdale

Actress, Singer, and Songwriter

This Gurl smiles all the time. She's full of energy and loves bright makeup, which completely suits her personality. She's totally cute and has a really strong sense of style. It shows!

LIKE THIS LOOK? I gave this same look to Christine in "Lime Light" (page 111). Instead of Christine's lime-colored liner, I softened Ashley's look by using a teal blue pencil along the upper and lower lash lines. Bronzer was also added to the apples of Ashley's cheeks.

Jinsol

Spirited and fiery, Jinsol really lights up a room. Her beauty stems from self-reliance, resourcefulness, and a belief in herself.

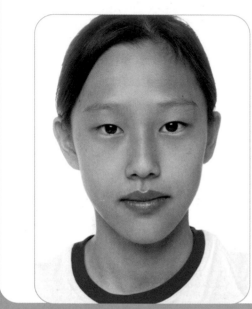

BEFORE: Jinsol has no spots whatsoever! I did choose to even out her skin tone just a bit, to brighten up dark circles under her eyes, and to lightly shape her eyebrows.

Tools
Toner
Moisturizer with SPF
Concealer
Translucent powder
Rose crème blush
Sheer berry lip gloss
Brow gel
Medium brown eyebrow pencil
Gold shimmer powder eye shadow
Lash curler
Black mascara

FLAWLESS FINISH

Get This Look

Step 1
Start with clean, prepped skin. Wash your face, then apply toner and a light moisturizer with SPF. Let the products soak into your skin for five minutes. Blot away any excess with a tissue.

Step 2
Apply concealer with your *ring* fingertip, that's the one next to your pinkie. Dab in the bottom and top inner corners of your eyes and below your eyes, out and over, or wherever you see blue, gray, or red. Blend down and out by tapping the concealer into place until there are no distinct lines. Rub any leftover concealer on any redness around your nostrils and on any spots.

Step 3
Set your concealer by lightly tapping translucent powder over it with a puff or a fluffy brush.

Step 4
Using your fingers, apply the blush on the apples of your cheeks, keeping the edges soft and blended.

Step 5
Sweep the gloss over your lips.

Step 6
Use the brush of your eyebrow gel to brush your eyebrows up and out. Fill in any gaps with the eyebrow pencil. Apply less than you think you should.

Step 7
Blend the eye shadow on your lids using a side-to-side motion, starting at the lash line and working your way up until just beneath your brow bone.

Step 8
Curl your lashes and apply one coat of mascara.

The Look: Clean and sweet. Ideal for school or a family dinner at your friend's house.

Why It's a Winner: The gold, rose, and berry warm up the natural yellow tones in Asian skin—bringing out the luscious!

What the Pros Say: "There was a time when Asian women wanted to change their eyes to look more Anglo. That's over! As a model scout, I look for exotic eyes!" —James Charles, Director of New Faces, L.A. Models agency

The Bigger Picture: Celebrate the way you *actually* look!

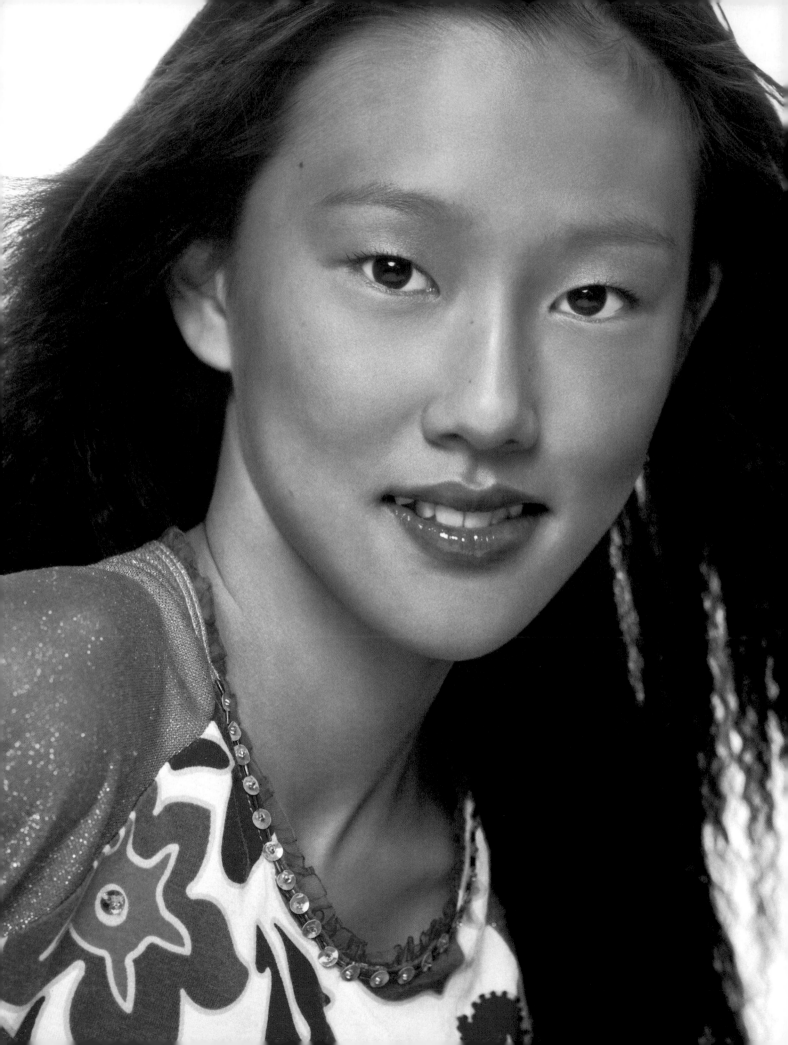

ISLE OF STYLE

The Look: A great festive party look that's super-soft.

Get This Look

Step 1
Start with clean, prepped skin. Wash your face, then apply toner and a light moisturizer with SPF. Let the products soak into your skin for five minutes. Blot away any excess with a tissue.

Step 2
Apply concealer with your *ring* fingertip, that's the one next to your pinkie. Dab in the bottom and top inner corners of your eyes and below your eyes, out and over, or wherever you see blue, gray, or red. Blend down and out by tapping the concealer into place until there are no distinct lines. Rub any leftover concealer on any redness around your nostrils and on any spots.

Step 3
Set your concealer by lightly tapping translucent powder over it with a puff or a fluffy brush.

Step 4
Lightly dust the blush on the apples of the cheeks and blend out toward the ears.

Step 5
Cover your lips with the gloss to really make your mouth pop!

Step 6
Use the brush of your eyebrow gel to brush your eyebrows up and out. Fill in any gaps with the eyebrow pencil. Apply less than you think you should.

Step 7
Dip your eye shadow brush in the shimmery gold eye shadow, flick off the excess, and then apply the product in the center of your lid, below the crease. Spread out the product in a side-to-side motion, from the lash line to just below your brow bone.

Step 8
Curl your lashes and apply one coat of mascara.

Why It's a Winner: This breezy look takes pink tones on Asian skin to the next level!

What the Pros Say: "She's beautiful, not only because of the way she looks but because she's proud of who she is." —Tracy Bayne, fashion photographer for Beyoncé Knowles

The Bigger Picture: There was a time when Asian, Anglo, and even African, Caribbean, and African-American Gurlz wanted to look lighter. Today, that beauty standard has gone out the window. Celebrate your natural skin tone!

Brit

This straight-A student is quiet and intuitive. She's also a champion horseback rider, she loves to volunteer, and she's a role model for her little sister. The future looks bright for this Gurl.

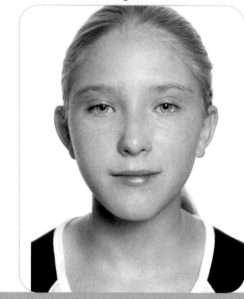

BEFORE: I chose to brighten the lines under Brit's eyes and shape her brows.

Tools
Toner
Tinted moisturizer with SPF
Concealer
Face/Translucent powder
Gold shimmer powder blush
Apricot lip gloss
Brow gel
Blonde eyebrow pencil
White shimmer crème eye shadow
Lash curler
Black mascara

prep skool

The Look: Perfect for the active Gurl . . . this look is fresh, clean, and natural.

Get This Look

Step 1
Start with clean, prepped skin. Wash your face, then apply toner. Let the product soak into your skin for five minutes.

Step 2
Using clean hands, apply a tinted moisturizer with SPF on your face. Start at the center and blend out toward the ends of the face. Be sure to blend down your neck. Notice how it evens out your skin tone?

Step 3
Apply concealer with your *ring* fingertip, that's the one next to your pinkie. Dab in the bottom and top inner corners of your eyes and below your eyes, out and over, or wherever you see blue, gray, or red. Blend down and out by tapping the concealer into place until there are no distinct lines. Rub any leftover concealer on any redness around your nostrils and on any spots.

Step 4
Set your concealer by lightly tapping translucent powder over it with a puff or a fluffy brush.

Step 5
Using a blush brush, apply the blush to the apples of your cheeks, keeping the edges soft and blended.

Step 6
Use a lip brush to apply the gloss over your lips.

Step 7
Use the brush of your eyebrow gel to brush your eyebrows up and out. Fill in any gaps with the eyebrow pencil. Apply less than you think you should.

Step 8
Lightly dab your lids with the white eye shadow. Using your finger, spread the product from side to side, starting at the lash line and working up to the crease. Stop there, but blend well at the edge so there won't be a hard line.

Step 9
Curl lashes and apply one coat of mascara to the *top* lashes only.

Jewel Staite

Actress

When beautiful Jewel told me her thoughts about the pressures of high school life, I was impressed—her message was so powerful and strong. It made me stop and think: Jewel is a perfect example of a Gurl who uses all of her smartz.

JEWEL SAYS

"In high school it's usually the scantily clad Gurlz who get the attention of the boys. It's hard to remember that not all attention is positive attention. I think having self-respect is more important than having a boyfriend."

Like This Look?
I gave this same look to Brittany in "Retro Glam" (page 52). Instead of going bright on the eyes, Jewel goes neutral with a medium brown pressed powder eye shadow, blended just above the crease.

get in your space

Surround yourself with things you love, whether that be music, pets, or just stuff that makes you feel good. Hook up your locker with photos of friends . . . rearrange your bedroom until you find what suits your style . . .

Then on days when you feel low, you'll have plenty of reminders of who you are and what makes you happy and you'll be back on track in no time!

zen again

Personal growth is not just for grown-ups! If you know you look great on the outside, but feel terrble on the inside, STOP and take time to figure out *why* you are feeling the way you do.

You gotta grow on the inside just like you are growing on the outside. How do you do it? If you spend 10 minutes a day doing your makeup, also spend 10 minutes working on your soul . . . by giving yourself props for the things that you do well.

Nicole

Nicole doesn't buy into the idea of typical beauty. And she doesn't rely on her looks to get her where she's going. To Nicole, being pretty is a blessing, not a card to play.

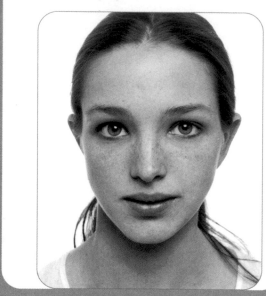

BEFORE: I covered up a couple of spots, brightened Nicole's under-eye area, evened out her complexion, and shaped her brows.

Tools
Toner
Tinted moisturizer with SPF
Concealer
Face/Translucent powder
Bright orange crème blush
Natural lip liner pencil in a shade just slightly darker than your lip tone
Rose lip gloss
Brow gel
Medium brown eyebrow pencil
Copper shimmer crème eye shadow
Lash curler
Black mascara

Fresh Face

the Look: Warm tones make this look ideal for a dinner out on the town.

Get This Look

Step 1

Start with clean, prepped skin. Wash your face, then apply toner. Let the product soak into your skin for five minutes.

Step 2

Using clean hands, rub a tinted moisturizer with SPF on your face. Start at the center and blend out toward the ends of the face. Be sure to blend down your neck.

Step 3

Apply concealer with your *ring* fingertip, that's the one next to your pinkie. Dab in the bottom and top inner corners of your eyes and below your eyes, out and over, or wherever you see blue, gray, or red. Blend down and out by tapping the concealer into place until there are no distinct lines. Rub any leftover concealer on any redness around your nostrils and on any spots.

Step 4

Set your tinted moisturizer and concealer by lightly dusting powder over the face with a puff or a big fluffy brush.

Step 5

Using your fingers, apply the blush on the apples of your cheeks, blending it out toward the ear only a little bit.

Step 6

Softly line along your natural lip line with the lip liner.

Step 7

Use your lip brush to apply the lip gloss. Blend your gloss and lip liner together.

Step 8

Use the brush of your eyebrow gel to brush your eyebrows up and out. Fill in any gaps with the eyebrow pencil. Apply less than you think you should.

Step 9

Wash the eye shadow all over your lids and blend up toward your brow bone.

Step 10

Curl your lashes and apply one coat of mascara.

Why It's a Winner: These rich colors really make Nicole's overall look brighter and sunnier.

What the Pros Say: Her *skin tone* is the strongest part of this look!" —Miles Haddad, celebrity hairstylist to LeAnn Rimes and Scarlett Johansson

The Bigger Picture: You may notice that the Glamour Gurlz look hardly ever calls for a lip liner. In this case it works, because the liner is natural. Liner is generally used with lipstick, and the Glamour Gurlz look is all about *gloss*.

the look: This is *the* look for a party, a dance, or anywhere you want to make a fun statement.

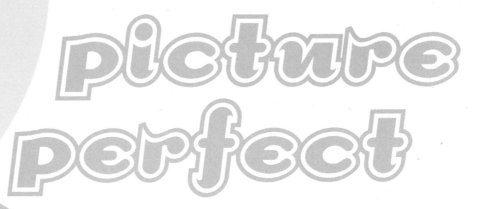

picture perfect

Tools
Toner
Tinted moisturizer with SPF
Concealer
Face/Translucent powder
Peach crème blush
Natural lip liner pencil in a shade just slightly darker than your lip tone
Sheer orange lip gloss
Brow gel
Medium brown eyebrow pencil
Lime green crème eye shadow
Lash curler
Black mascara

Get This Look

Step 1
Start with clean, prepped skin. Wash your face, then apply toner. Let the product soak into your skin for five minutes.

Step 2
Using clean hands, rub a tinted moisturizer with SPF on your face. Start at the center and blend out toward the ends of the face. Be sure to blend down your neck.

Step 3
Apply concealer with your *ring* fingertip, that's the one next to your pinkie. Dab in the bottom and top inner corners of your eyes and below your eyes, out and over, or wherever you see blue, gray, or red. Blend down and out by tapping the concealer into place until there are no distinct lines. Rub any leftover concealer on any redness around your nostrils and on any spots.

Step 4
Set your tinted moisturizer and concealer by lightly dusting powder over the face with a puff or a big fluffy brush.

Step 5
Using your fingers, apply the blush across the apples of your cheeks, blending it out toward your ears.

Step 6
Softly line along your natural lip line with the lip liner.

Step 7
Use your lip brush to apply the lip gloss. Blend the gloss and lip liner together.

Step 8
Use the brush of your eyebrow gel to brush your eyebrows up and out. Fill in any gaps with the eyebrow pencil. Apply less than you think you should.

Step 9
Wash the lime eye shadow all over the lid and blend it just to the crease of your eye.

Step 10
Curl your lashes and apply one coat of mascara.

Why It's a Winner: This unexpected color combination of orange and lime is eye-catching and beautiful at the same time.

What the Pros Say: "This look is fierce! Look at those eyes! Amazing!" —Crosby Carter, beauty industry agent

The Bigger Picture: Any time you draw attention to your eyes, either with makeup or with your natural gaze, you *draw in* the attention of those around you.

Alexis

Alexis knows who she is: She's definitely a leader with her own strong personal style.

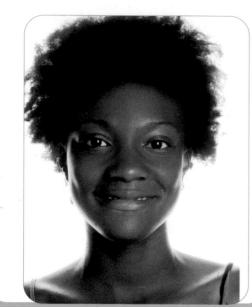

BEFORE: I concealed Alexis's few spots and a bit of darkness under her eyes. I also chose to shape her brows.

Tools
Toner
Moisturizer with SPF
Concealer
Face/Translucent powder
Amber crème blush
Caramel lip gloss
Brow gel
Dark brown eyebrow pencil
Soft black powder eye shadow
Lash curler
Black mascara

all eyes on me

Get This Look

Step 1
Start with clean, prepped skin. Wash your face, then apply toner and a light moisturizer with SPF. Let the products soak into your skin for five minutes. Blot away any excess with a tissue.

Step 2
Apply concealer with your *ring* fingertip, that's the one next to your pinkie. Dab in the bottom and top inner corners of your eyes and below your eyes, out and over, or wherever you see blue, gray, or red. Blend down and out by tapping the concealer into place until there are no distinct lines. Rub any leftover concealer on any redness around your nostrils and on any spots.

Step 3
Set your concealer by lightly tapping translucent powder over it with a puff or a fluffy brush.

Step 4
Using your fingers, apply the blush across your cheekbones, blending out toward your ears.

Step 5
Sweep on the lip gloss.

Step 6
Use the brush of your eyebrow gel to brush your eyebrows up and out. Fill in any gaps with the eyebrow pencil. Apply less than you think you should.

Step 7
Blend eye shadow on your lid starting at the lash line and working your way up to the crease, and stop there. Apply a soft line along the bottom of the lashes and blend so there are no hard lines.

Step 8
Curl your lashes and apply one coat of mascara.

The LOOK: Her beautiful skin is flawless, yet her eyes are the star here. By keeping all of the makeup neutral, I let her eyes take center stage with some smudged liner.

Why It's a Winner: This makeup makes her look polished and put together.

What the Pros Say: "Being pretty is only one attribute; this Gurl has that and a whole lot more!" —Peter Osegueda, celebrity wardrobe stylist to Nicole Richie

The Bigger Picture: No one makes her mark without taking a risk and putting herself out there. Make a difference.

Ky

Ky is a true nonconformist. The president of her class, Ky has the smartz to understand that popularity isn't everything. She finds her confidence in helping others, rooting for the underdog, and making genuine connections with genuine people.

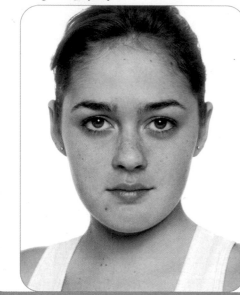

BEFORE: Ky tends to get dark circles under her eyes and a bit of skin discoloration. Our aim was to even out her skin tone without covering up the pretty freckles around her nose. Another great thing about Ky's skin? No visible pores!

Tools
Toner
Moisturizer with SPF
Concealer
Face/Translucent powder
Rose powder blush
Berry lip gloss
Brow gel
Medium brown eyebrow pencil
Light bronze shimmer powder eye shadow
Lash curler
Black mascara

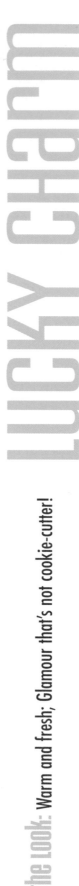

LUCKY CHARM

The look: Warm and fresh; Glamour that's not cookie-cutter!

Get This Look

Step 1
Start with clean, prepped skin. Wash your face, then apply toner and a light moisturizer with SPF. Let the products soak into your skin for five minutes. Blot away any excess with a tissue.

Step 2
Apply concealer with your *ring* fingertip, that's the one next to your pinkie. Dab in the bottom and top inner corners of your eyes and below your eyes, out and over, or wherever you see blue, gray, or red. Blend down and out by tapping the concealer into place until there are no distinct lines. Rub any leftover concealer on any redness around your nostrils and on any spots.

Step 3
Set your concealer by lightly tapping translucent powder over it with a puff or a fluffy brush.

Step 4
Dust the blush on the apples of your cheeks and blend out toward your ears.

Step 5
With a lip brush, apply the gloss to define your mouth.

Step 6
Use the brush of your eyebrow gel to brush your eyebrows up and out. Fill in any gaps with the eyebrow pencil. Apply less than you think you should.

Step 7
Wash the eye shadow all over the lids and blend up toward the brow.

Step 8
Curl your lashes and apply one coat of mascara.

SCHLIPTIP: Why so little coverage here? Ky has the cutest freckles on her nose and I want to show them off!

Why It's a Winner: Bronze and berry bring out the warm tones in Ky's skin.

What the Pros Say: As a hairstylist, I know that when a Gurl pulls her hair away from her face, she's showing confidence. I think the way she looks on the outside comes from how she feels on the inside . . . confident!" —Ken Pavés, celebrity hairstylist to Jessica Simpson and Eva Longoria

The Bigger Picture: What does the natural look really mean? It's simply shorthand for makeup that looks like you are not wearing any. The way you look on your happiest days without even trying.

pretty baby

The look: Cool lavender colors make this look fresh and clean.

Tools
Toner
Moisturizer with SPF
Concealer
Face/Translucent powder
Baby pink crème blush
Sheer pink lip gloss
Brow gel
Medium brown eyebrow pencil
Light lavender crème shimmer eye shadow
Lash curler
Black mascara

Get This Look

Step 1
Start with clean, prepped skin. Wash your face, then apply toner, and a light moisturizer with SPF. Let the products soak into your skin for five minutes. Blot away any excess with a tissue.

Step 2
Apply concealer with your *ring* fingertip, that's the one next to your pinkie. Dab in the bottom and top inner corners of your eyes and below your eyes, out and over, or wherever you see blue, gray, or red. Blend down and out by tapping the concealer into place until there are no distinct lines. Rub any leftover concealer on any redness around your nostrils and on any spots.

Step 3
Set your concealer by lightly tapping translucent powder over it with a puff or a fluffy brush.

Step 4
Using your fingers, wash the blush on the apples of the cheeks. Be sure to blend up toward your ears.

Step 5
Apply your gloss using a lip brush.

Step 6
Use the brush of your eyebrow gel to brush your eyebrows up and out. Fill in any gaps with the eyebrow pencil. Apply less than you think you should.

Step 7
Wash the eye shadow all over the lids and blend up toward the brow bone.

Step 8
Curl your lashes and apply one coat of mascara.

SCHLIPTIP ON COVERING BEAUTY MARKS: Covering moles and beauty marks is easy. But remember, it's not necessary! After all, they're called *beauty* marks for a reason. If you do want to cover, simply take the same concealer you would use under your eyes and spot it on your mole *before* your tinted moisturizer.

Why It's a Winner: Lavender and plum will always make green eyes *more* green—these colors really make them pop!

What the Pros Say: "She looks like she'd be the nicest Gurl in school. Friendly, talkative, popular, but still so nice." —Enzo Angileri, celebrity hairstylist to Charlize Theron

The Bigger Picture: When you have a distinctive feature like freckles, use your makeup to *highlight* that signature look—like super-model Cindy Crawford does with her mole. Glamour Gurlz show off what they got.

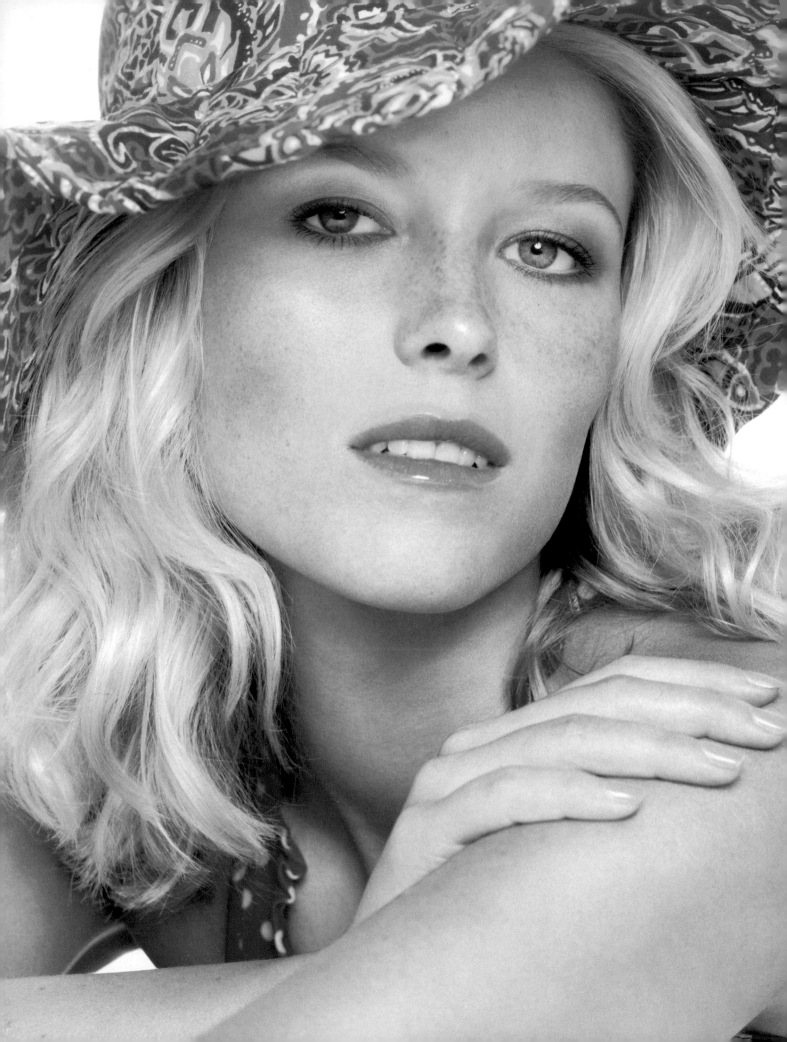

Kiera Chaplin

Actress

Kiera is not only beautiful, but she is also very self-assured and relaxed. There is a modern edge to her regal looks. Her focus? Work on your inner beauty; the rest will fall into place.

LIKE THIS LOOK? I gave this same look to Christine in "Boho, Baby!" (page 108). Kiera claims this look as her own with a smudge of brown pressed powder eye shadow along her lower lash line.

CITY pretty

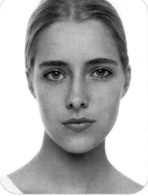

Jessica

Jessica has an inner light that shines through, making her all the more beautiful. Ask her what she's all about and she'll say: keeping it real, thinking for herself, and following her heart.

BEFORE: I brightened up her eyes and trimmed and shaped her brows.

The Look: This dressy look is great for going out on the town with your Gurlz . . . or your guy!

Tools
Toner
Tinted moisturizer with SPF
Concealer
Face/Translucent powder
Pink powder blush
Shiny pink lip gloss
Brow gel
Blonde eyebrow pencil
Black kohl eyeliner pencil
Cotton swab
Lash curler
Black mascara

Get This Look

Step 1
Start with clean, prepped skin. Wash your face, then apply toner. Let the product soak into your skin for five minutes.

Step 2
Using clean hands, rub a tinted moisturizer on your face. Start at the center and blend out toward the ends of the face. Be sure to blend down your neck.

Step 3
Apply concealer with your *ring* fingertip, that's the one next to your pinkie. Dab in the bottom and top inner corners of your eyes and below your eyes, out and over, or wherever you see blue, gray, or red. Blend down and out by tapping the concealer into place until there are no distinct lines. Rub any leftover concealer on any redness around your nostrils and on any spots.

Step 4
Set your tinted moisturizer and concealer by lightly dusting powder over the face with a puff or a big fluffy brush.

Step 5
Wash the blush very lightly over the apples of your cheeks.

Step 6
Using your lip brush, apply some lip gloss.

Step 7
Use the brush of your eyebrow gel to brush your eyebrows up and out. Fill in any gaps with the eyebrow pencil. Apply less than you think you should.

Step 8
Line all the way around the outside of your eye with the eyeliner. Then line all around the *inside* of your eye. Finish off by smudging the outside liner with a clean shadow brush or a cotton swab.

Step 9
Curl your lashes and apply *two* coats of mascara.

Why It's a Winner:

This look has star power! The smoky liner really makes her blue eyes pop. So pretty!

What the Pros Say:

"This Gurl is happy to be who she is and it shows!" —Peter Osegueda, wardrobe stylist to Nicole Richie

The Bigger Picture:

Highlighting your eyes with eyeliner *does* draw attention to them, but you won't hold anyone's gaze if you don't actively *use* your eyes to communicate what you're trying to say. Regardless of what's on them, eyes *are* power. Use them.

Lily

Self-confidence and attitude give Lily her *je ne sais quoi.* Her own Gurl inside and out, Lily trusts herself enough to take risks and gives herself room to spread her wings and fly.

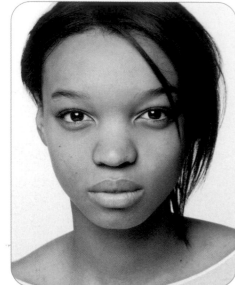

BEFORE: Lily's look only called for a bit of lightening under her eyes and a shaping of her brows.

Tools
Toner
Tinted moisturizer with SPF
Concealer
Face/Translucent powder
Soft pink pressed powder blush
Sheer pink lip gloss
Brow gel
Dark brown eyebrow pencil
Shimmery plum powder eye shadow
Lash curler
Black mascara

crazy cute!

The Look: Wear this makeup during the day and then touch it up to keep going into night. It's the ultimate, versatile Glamour Gurl look!

Get This Look

Step 1
Start with clean, prepped skin. Wash your face, then apply toner. Let the product soak into your skin for five minutes.

Step 2
Using clean hands, apply a tinted moisturizer on your face. Start at the center and blend out toward the ends of the face. Be sure to blend down your neck.

Step 3
Apply concealer with your *ring* fingertip, that's the one next to your pinkie. Dab in the bottom and top inner corners of your eyes and below your eyes, out and over, or wherever you see blue, gray, or red. Blend down and out by tapping the concealer into place until there are no distinct lines. Rub any leftover concealer on any redness around your nostrils and on any spots.

Step 4
Set your concealer by lightly tapping translucent powder over it with a puff or a fluffy brush.

Step 5
Use a blush brush to apply the blush to the apples of your cheeks, keeping the edges soft and blended.

Step 6
Use a lip brush to apply your lip gloss.

Step 7
Use the brush of your eyebrow gel to brush your eyebrows up and out. Fill in any gaps with the eyebrow pencil. Apply less than you think you should.

Step 8
Apply a thin swipe of the plum eye shadow to your lash line, then work it in up to the crease and blend well.

Step 9
Curl lashes and apply one coat of mascara to the top lashes only.

Why It's a Winner: Plum shades bring out eye color!

What the Pros Say: "There is no stopping this Gurl. She looks confident and determined. A no-nonsense kind of Gurl." —Jenny Cho, celebrity hairstylist to Ashlee Simpson and Michelle Trachtenberg

The Bigger Picture: It doesn't matter what eye color you have, as long as you highlight it in a way that brings out its best!

Brie Larson

Actress, Singer, and Songwriter

When I heard the song "Ugly" and then saw the gorgeous Gurl who wrote it, I couldn't believe those words and thoughts came from such a young beauty. Brie Larson is incredible inside and out. I knew that if I could relate to her words, many of you would relate as well. We have all experienced moments where we feel "less-than." It is important for you to know that they are just thoughts and not the truth about you!

UGLY

by Brie Larson

My insides are turning inside out
Leaving my heart, my flaws all hanging out
What's so interesting about little ol' me?
All I see is so ordinary
I can't look at myself
I can't find nothing special hiding in me
I can't look in myself
You tell me it's there to see but all I see is so . . . ugly.

Like This Look? I gave this same look to Mia in "Indigo Gurl" (page 162). I swapped out Mia's blue for a beautiful emerald-green liquid eyeliner.

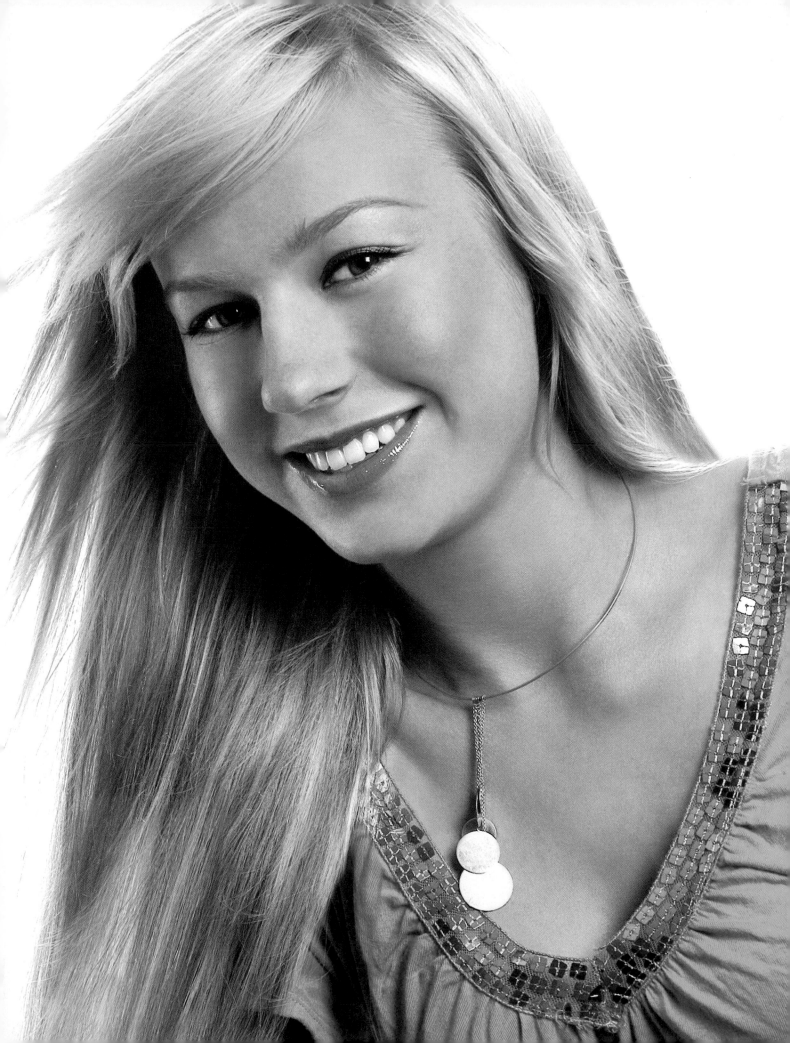

what's your fla'va?

Jessica Simpson is beautiful. Few Gurlz would disagree with that. But so is Beyoncé—and they look nothing alike. In fact, all the Gurlz in this book are beautiful, but in totally different ways. They each have their own **FLA'VA**.

When it comes to the pretty list, there's room for everyone!

drama-rama!

Ever feel like there's way too much drama in your life? Let me tell you: Tears happen . . . and that's *okay*. So you get mad, get sad, and move on. Take charge of your life. It is YOURS to live!

Every day is a new opportunity waiting to happen just for you!

Margarita

This aspiring writer has many layers. She's an old soul with a pixie face. Watch out for this Gurl; she's going places!

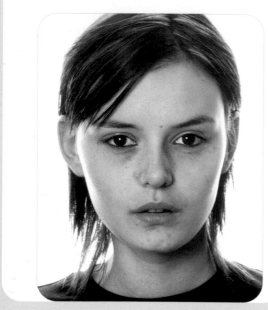

BEFORE: Margarita's dramatic looks tend to give her dark circles under her eyes. She has a bit of an uneven skin tone and a couple of spots. I fixed these and also chose to clean and shape her eyebrows.

Tools
Toner
Tinted moisturizer with SPF
Concealer
Face/Translucent powder
Warm pink powder blush
Golden shimmer powder
Sparkly, peach-colored lip gloss
Brow gel
Medium brown eyebrow pencil
Mint-green pressed powder shimmer
eye shadow
Brown kohl eyeliner pencil
Lash curler
Black mascara

Pixie Dust

The Look: Bright and happy, ready for a day of fun and adventure!

Get This Look

Step 1
Start with clean, prepped skin. Wash your face, then apply toner. Let the product soak into your skin for five minutes.

Step 2
Apply tinted moisturizer with SPF in the same tone as your skin. Blend well all over. Don't forget to draw the product down below your jaw line.

Step 3
Dab concealer in the bottom and top inner corners of your eyes and below your eyes, or wherever you see blue, gray, or red. Blend down and out by tapping the concealer into place until there are no distinct lines. Rub any leftover concealer on any redness around your nostrils and on any spots.

Step 4
Set your concealer by lightly tapping translucent powder over it with a puff or a fluffy brush.

Step 5
Use your brush to dust the blush on the apples of your cheeks and just below your cheekbones. Then apply the golden shimmer powder along the highest part of the cheekbone for instant Glamour.

Step 6
Cover your lips with the gloss to make your lips really stand out.

Step 7
Use the brush of your eyebrow gel to brush your eyebrows up and out. Fill in any gaps with the eyebrow pencil. Apply less than you think you should.

Step 8
Blend the eye shadow on your lids, starting at the lash line and working up to the crease. Do not apply it above the crease.

Step 9
Using the eyeliner pencil, line close to the lashes on both the top and the bottom.

Step 10
Curl your lashes and apply one coat of mascara to the *top* lashes only.

Why It's a Winner: The mint-green color really brings out the pink in her cheeks.

What the Pros Say: "You always think boys like long hair, but in Margarita's case, her short cut puts it all together!" —James Charles, Director of New Faces, L.A. Models agency

The Bigger Picture: How will you ever know if something fits unless you try it on? Have the guts to take a risk. Introduce yourself to someone new, sit in the front row. Try a new look. Sometimes you might think you made a mistake. But mistakes are really just lessons you needed to learn. You might discover the very thing that rocks your world.

urban edge

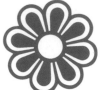

The Look: A deep, hard edge or smoky eye that's all drama, all the time, for a fun night out with the Gurlz or a concert.

SCHLIPTIP: If you want that smudged, smoky look, use a softer kohl pencil. Apply it to your eye and smudge with a cotton swab or your eye-shadow brush. Keep in mind that eyeliner is difficult to clean from your brush.

Tools
Toner
Tinted moisturizer with SPF
Concealer
Face/Translucent powder
Pale pink powder blush
Pink lip gloss
Brow gel
Medium brown eyebrow pencil
Jet-black kohl eyeliner pencil
Lash curler
Black mascara

Get This Look

Step 1
Start with clean, prepped skin. Wash your face, then apply toner. Let the product soak into your skin for five minutes.

Step 2
Using clean hands, apply a tinted moisturizer with SPF on your face. Start at the center and blend out toward the ends of the face. Be sure to blend down your neck.

Step 3
Apply concealer with your *ring* fingertip, that's the one next to your pinkie. Dab in the bottom and top inner corners of your eyes and below your eyes, out and over, or wherever you see blue, gray, or red. Blend down and out by tapping the concealer into place until there are no distinct lines. Rub any leftover concealer on any redness around your nostrils and on any spots.

Step 4
Set your concealer by lightly tapping translucent powder over it with a puff or a fluffy brush.

Step 5
Dust the blush onto the apples of your cheeks and blend high onto the cheekbones.

Step 6
Cover your lips with the pink gloss for a natural glow.

Step 7
Use the brush of your eyebrow gel to brush your eyebrows up and out. Fill in any gaps with the eyebrow pencil. Apply less than you think you should.

Step 8
Use the kohl pencil to line the upper and lower lash line with a thick stroke. Make one more stroke along the lower, inside edge. No eye shadow necessary for this look.

Step 9
Curl your lashes and apply one coat of mascara to top lashes only.

Why It's a Winner:

Margarita has incredibly expressive eyes. This look shows them off in a soft way that's not too Goth.

What the Pros Say:

"Makeup should be fun—just another way to feel better about yourself—not a mask to hide behind." —Kate Dimmock, fashion magazine director

The Bigger Picture: By

pairing a really dramatic eye treatment with simple—almost colorless!—cheeks and lips, you can enjoy the most hard-core looks while still being pretty.

Elsa

She's a star and doesn't even know it yet! Elsa's determined and focused with the grace of a southern belle. At fourteen, she's just beginning to tap into her own unique style.

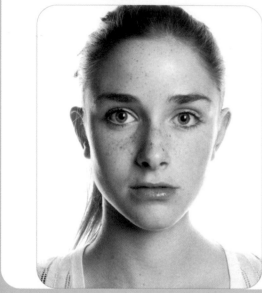

BEFORE: I lightened just under Elsa's eyes and cleaned up her brows.

Tools
Toner
Moisturizer with SPF
Concealer
Face/Translucent powder
Rose crème blush
Sheer pink lip gloss
Brow gel
Light brown eyebrow pencil
Lash curler
Black mascara

rising star

Get This Look

Step 1
Start with clean, prepped skin. Wash your face, then apply toner and a light moisturizer with SPF. Let the products soak into your skin for five minutes. Blot away any excess with a tissue.

Step 2
Apply concealer with your *ring* fingertip, that's the one next to your pinkie. Dab in the bottom and top inner corners of your eyes and below your eyes, out and over, or wherever you see blue, gray, or red. Blend down and out by tapping the concealer into place until there are no distinct lines. Rub any leftover concealer on any redness around your nostrils and on any spots.

Step 3
Set your concealer by lightly tapping translucent powder over it with a puff or a fluffy brush.

Step 4
Using your fingers, apply the blush to the apples of your cheeks, keeping the edges soft and blended.

Step 5
Sweep the gloss over your lips.

Step 6
Use the brush of your eyebrow gel to brush your eyebrows up and out. Fill in any gaps with the eyebrow pencil. Apply less than you think you should.

Step 7
No eye shadow for this look!

Step 8
Curl your lashes and apply one coat of mascara to both your top *and* bottom lashes.

The Look: This treatment's focus on the lashes draws you into her eyes . . . one of her best features!

Why It's a Winner: Another great option for the natural-wonder look that also shows off Elsa's freckles!

What the Pros Say: "Her eyes are the 'stars' in this picture. Attractive, alluring, and amazing!" —Jenny Cho, celebrity hairstylist to Ashlee Simpson and Michelle Trachtenberg

The Bigger Picture: The eyes have it. Always. You'll know when you've captured a new school friend's imagination if he or she can't stop watching you!

Mia

She's a sweet Gurl with big dreams. Mia's blessed with gorgeous skin and mile-long lashes, and she loves playing them up with makeup.

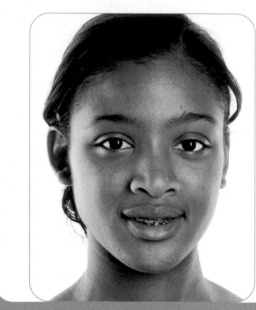

BEFORE: Mia has a few spots that I chose to cover. I also evened out her skin tone and brightened the area underneath her eyes.

Tools
Toner
Tinted moisturizer with SPF
Concealer
Face/Translucent powder
Peach pressed powder blush
Clear lip gloss with flecks of glitter
Brow gel
Light brown eyebrow pencil
Silver shimmer powder eye shadow
Lash curler
Black mascara

quick silver

The Look: Glam up your eyes with a strong silver eye shadow.

Get This Look

Step 1
Start with clean, prepped skin. Wash your face, then apply toner. Let the product soak into your skin for five minutes.

Step 2
Using clean hands, apply a tinted moisturizer with SPF on your face. Start at the center and blend out toward the ends of the face. Be sure to blend down your neck.

Step 3
Apply concealer with your *ring* fingertip, that's the one next to your pinkie. Dab in the bottom and top inner corners of your eyes and below your eyes, out and over, or wherever you see blue, gray, or red. Blend down and out by tapping the concealer into place until there are no distinct lines. Rub any leftover concealer on any redness around your nostrils and on any spots.

Step 4
Set your concealer by lightly tapping translucent powder over it with a puff or a fluffy brush.

Step 5
Lightly dust the blush on the apples of your cheeks and blend out toward the ears.

Step 6
Cover your lips with the glitter-flecked gloss for a little something new.

Step 7
Use the brush of your eyebrow gel to brush your eyebrows up and out. Fill in any gaps with the eyebrow pencil. Apply less than you think you should.

Step 8
Blend the eye shadow onto your lids, starting at the lash line and working your way up almost to the brow bone.

Step 9
Curl your lashes and apply one coat of mascara to the *top* lashes only.

Why It's a Winner: Solid silver on the eyes is a rich, powerful look that's still fun enough for a night out with your Gurlz.

What the Pros Say: "You can see that she has something going on behind those eyes." —Andrew Matusik, fashion photographer for Hilary Duff

The Bigger Picture: Put yourself out there, Gurl. You've got to believe you're *that* great. Only when *you* get behind this message, can you expect others to follow.

indigo gurl

The Look: Wear this bold look to the movies, a concert, or any place where you want to look creative and colorful.

SCHLIPTIP: LESS IS MORE! Before you apply *anything*, cut the amount of product in half! It's easy to add more, but super-time-consuming to start over!

Tools
Toner
Tinted moisturizer with SPF
Concealer
Face/Translucent powder
Pink pressed powder blush
Clear lip gloss
Brow gel
Light brown eyebrow pencil
Brown shimmer powder eye shadow
Electric-blue liquid eyeliner
Lash curler
Black mascara

Get This Look

Step 1
Start with clean, prepped skin. Wash your face, then apply toner. Let the product soak into your skin for five minutes.

Step 2
Using clean hands, apply a tinted moisturizer with SPF on your face. Start at the center and blend out toward the ends of the face. Be sure to blend down your neck.

Step 3
Apply concealer with your *ring* fingertip, that's the one next to your pinkie. Dab in the bottom and top inner corners of your eyes and below your eyes, out and over, or wherever you see blue, gray, or red. Blend down and out by tapping the concealer into place until there are no distinct lines. Rub any leftover concealer on any redness around your nostrils and on any spots.

Step 4
Set your concealer by lightly tapping translucent powder over it with a puff or a fluffy brush.

Step 5
Using your brush, lightly dust the blush on the apples of the cheeks and blend out toward the ears.

Step 6
Cover your lips with the clear gloss for a subtle effect. The drama comes from the eyes for this look and you don't want the two to clash.

Step 7
Use the brush of your eyebrow gel to brush your eyebrows up and out. Fill in any gaps with the eyebrow pencil. Apply less than you think you should.

Step 8
Blend the eye shadow onto your lids, starting at the lash line and working your way up almost to the brow bone.

Step 9
Apply a line of liquid eyeliner along the top lashes only. Extend it out past the edge of the eye and wing the line up slightly.

Step 10
Curl your lashes and apply one coat of mascara to the *top* lashes only.

Why It's a Winner: The blue brings out Mia's gorgeous skin and eyes; the soft nude lips provide balance.

What the Pros Say: "She looks so beautiful in these colors, but then, this Gurl seems like she's all about the unexpected." —Luc Brinker, model agent for Wilhelmina Models

The Bigger Picture: Blue is one of those makeup treatments that must be used sparingly, but it is a definite classic, particularly with gorgeous dark skin.

The Look: Daring, strong party wear that pairs beautifully with accessories.

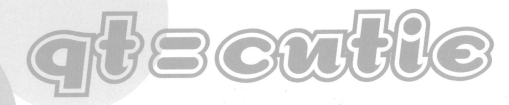

Tools

Toner
Tinted moisturizer with SPF
Concealer
Face/Translucent powder
Coral crème blush
Sheer pink lip gloss
Brow gel
Light brown eyebrow pencil
Cocoa-brown shimmer pressed eye shadow
Lash curler
Black mascara

Get This Look

Step 1

Start with clean, prepped skin. Wash your face, then apply toner. Let the product soak into your skin for five minutes.

Step 2

Using clean hands, apply a tinted moisturizer with SPF on your face. Start at the center and blend out toward the ends of the face. Be sure to blend down your neck.

Step 3

Apply concealer with your *ring* fingertip, that's the one next to your pinkie. Dab in the bottom and top inner corners of your eyes and below your eyes, out and over, or wherever you see blue, gray, or red. Blend down and out by tapping the concealer into place until there are no distinct lines. Rub any leftover concealer on any redness around your nostrils and on any spots.

Step 4

Set your concealer by lightly tapping translucent powder over it with a puff or a fluffy brush.

Step 5

Use your fingers to apply a small dab of blush on the apples of the cheeks and blend out toward the ears.

Step 6

Cover your lips with the sheer gloss for a natural effect.

Step 7

Use the brush of your eyebrow gel to brush your eyebrows up and out. Fill in any gaps with the eyebrow pencil. Apply less than you think you should.

Step 8

Blend the eye shadow onto the lids, starting at the lash line and working your way up just to the crease.

Step 9

Curl your lashes and apply one coat of mascara to the top lashes only.

Why It's a Winner: This cocoa-brown shadow turns the "Quick Silver" (page 160) look on its head: same technique but totally different effect.

What the Pros Say: "She looks strong here, but also really approachable. That's tough to pull off." —Peter Osegueda, wardrobe stylist for Nicole Richie

The Bigger Picture: Cocoa brown is dark enough to create drama, but it doesn't look as hard as black eye shadow. And let's face it, what pretty Gurl ever wants to look *totally* hard? Even gorgeous Goth or Straight-Edge Gurlz blend their makeup.

Lily B

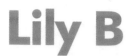

This Gurl knows who she is. She takes risks and is true to herself.

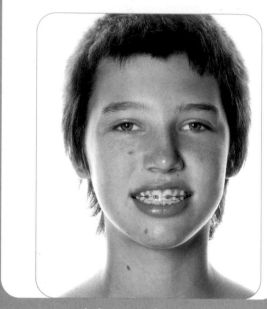

BEFORE: Lily has just a few spots on her face, a bit of uneven skin tone, and dark circles underneath her eyes. I fixed these and also cleaned up her eyebrows and, at her request, covered up her mole.

Tools
Toner
Tinted moisturizer with SPF
Concealer
Face/Translucent powder
Pink shimmer powder blush
Rose lip gloss
Brow gel
Light brown eyebrow pencil
Shimmer gold crème eye shadow
Lash curler
Black mascara

Campus Crisp

The Look: Together and getting stuff done . . . this Gurl knows what she wants and how to get it!

Get This Look

Step 1
Start with clean, prepped skin. Wash your face, then apply toner. Let the product soak into your skin for five minutes.

Step 2
Using clean hands, apply a tinted moisturizer on your face. Start at the center and blend out toward the ends of the face. Be sure to blend down your neck.

Step 3
Apply concealer with your *ring* fingertip, that's the one next to your pinkie. Dab in the bottom and top inner corners of your eyes and below your eyes, out and over, or wherever you see blue, gray, or red. Blend down and out by tapping the concealer into place until there are no distinct lines. Rub any leftover concealer on any redness around your nostrils and on any spots.

Step 4
Set your concealer by lightly tapping translucent powder over it with a puff or a fluffy brush.

Step 5
Apply the blush, but *only* on the apples of your cheeks.

Step 6
Apply the lip gloss over the lips.

Step 7
Use the brush of your eyebrow gel to brush your eyebrows up and out. Fill in any gaps with the eyebrow pencil. Apply less than you think you should.

Step 8
With your finger, apply the eye shadow to your lash line. Blend up using a side-to-side motion, but just to the crease.

Step 9
Curl your lashes and apply one coat of mascara to the top lashes only.

Why It's a Winner: This look highlights Lily's bright round cheeks! A major beauty asset!

What the Pros Say: "I always look for moles, gaps in teeth, and other interesting marks on my new models. These small 'perfections' are the difference between a pretty Gurl and a working model!"—James Charles, Director of New Faces, L.A. Models agency

The Bigger Picture: I covered Lily B's mole because she wanted to learn how to cover beauty marks the way the pros do. But the truth is that moles always look better when you show them off, or even highlight them by making the beauty mark darker.

glitter glam

the look: A fun glitter look that makes ordinary glitter treatments look *so two years ago.* It's a party in a jar!

SCHLIPTIP ON USING GLITTER: Be sure to buy glitter gel designed for use around your eyes! Otherwise the glitter might have sharp edges that will get into your eyes and irritate or damage them!

Tools
Toner
Tinted moisturizer with SPF
Concealer
Face/Translucent powder
Pink shimmer powder blush
Pink lip gloss
Brow gel
Light brown eyebrow pencil
Pink glitter gel for eyes

Get This Look

Step 1
Start with clean, prepped skin. Wash your face, then apply toner. Let the products soak into your skin for five minutes.

Step 2
Using clean hands, apply a tinted moisturizer with SPF on your face. Start at the center and blend out toward the ends of the face. Be sure to blend down your neck.

Step 3
Apply concealer with your *ring* fingertip, that's the one next to your pinkie. Dab in the bottom and top inner corners of your eyes and below your eyes, out and over, or wherever you see blue, gray, or red. Blend down and out by tapping the concealer into place until there are no distinct lines. Rub any leftover concealer on any redness around your nostrils and on any spots.

Step 4
Set your concealer by lightly tapping translucent powder over it with a puff or a fluffy brush.

Step 5
Use your brush to whisk on the blush on the apples of your cheeks.

Step 6
Apply the lip gloss over the lips.

Step 7
Use the brush of your eyebrow gel to brush your eyebrows up and out. Fill in any gaps with the eyebrow pencil. Apply less than you think you should.

Step 8
Using your finger, blend the glitter gel onto your lid. Begin along the lash line and blend all the way up to your brow. To avoid your glitter sticking and flaking, do one eye at a time and allow the glitter gel to dry before opening your eye and continuing. Why not use a brush? Glitter gel spreads best with your finger or a sponge-tip applicator.

Step 9
No mascara was used for this look, to keep the focus on the glitter.

Why It's a Winner:

Glitter adds a little something; this treatment uses glitter in a more sophisticated way.

What the Pros Say:

"I love her makeup! It's soo beautiful. I love the sparkle."
—Shinko Iura, celebrity wardrobe stylist to Claire Danes and Taryn Manning

The Bigger Picture:

Moles are usually harmless collections of pigmented cells on your skin, or *melanocytes*. Most of us have about ten to forty moles! Most moles show up by age twenty, and may actually fade away as you get older. It's really important to remember what your moles look like and tell your doctor if they change color or shape.

Andrea Bowen

Actress, Singer, Dancer

Beautiful Andrea Bowen is all about family and making everyone she meets feel as if they are a part of it. To Andrea beauty is all about unconditional love for others!

ANDREA SAYS

"Beauty to me is a lot more than the way you look on the outside. Confidence and generosity are what beauty is to me. You can see those traits in a person immediately, and when someone exudes those qualities, she is gorgeous!"

LIKE THIS LOOK? I gave this same look to Elsa in "Rising Star" (page 158). The only difference here is I added a lavender shimmer eye shadow on her top lid and on the bottom of her eye, right under her lashes.

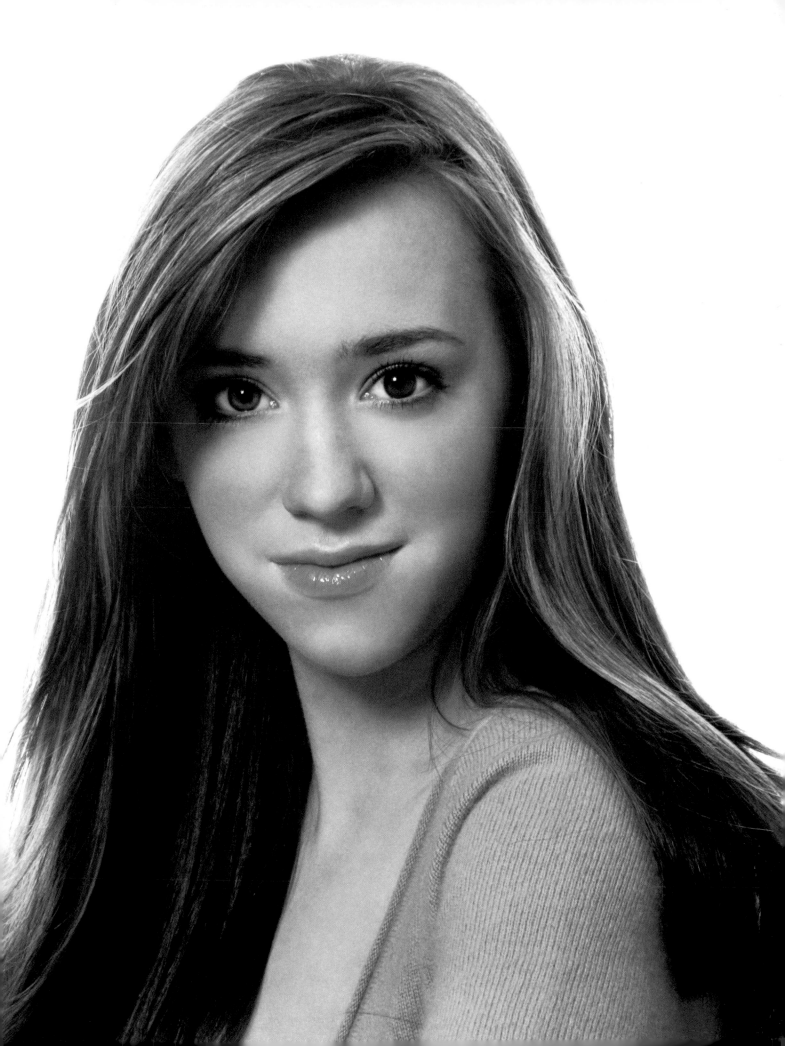

Piper

This Gurl's got edge to her style. She's strong in her beliefs, and doesn't follow the pack. Instead of following trends, she sets them!

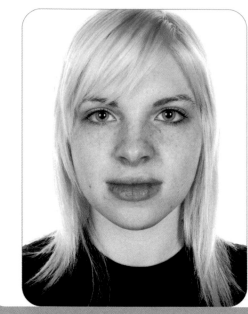

BEFORE: I chose to lighten underneath her eyes, even out her skin tone, moisturize her beautiful (but chapped!) full lips, cover up spots, and shape her brows.

Tools
Toner
Tinted moisturizer with SPF
Concealer
Face/Translucent powder
Pink cheek stain
Pink lip gloss
Brow gel
Blonde eyebrow pencil
Lash curler
Black mascara

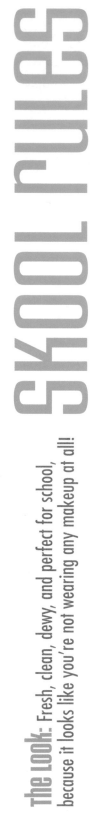

skool rules

The Look: Fresh, clean, dewy, and perfect for school, because it looks like you're not wearing any makeup at all!

Get This Look

Step 1
Start with clean, prepped skin. Wash your face, then apply toner. Let the product soak into your skin for five minutes.

Step 2
Using clean hands, apply a tinted moisturizer with SPF on your face. Start at the center and blend out toward the ends of the face. Be sure to blend down your neck.

Step 3
Apply concealer with your *ring* fingertip, that's the one next to your pinkie. Dab in the bottom and top inner corners of your eyes and below your eyes, out and over, or wherever you see blue, gray, or red. Blend down and out by tapping the concealer into place until there are no distinct lines. Rub any leftover concealer on any redness around your nostrils and on any spots.

Step 4
Set your concealer under your eyes by lightly tapping translucent powder over it with a puff or a fluffy brush.

Step 5
Ready for some color? Use your fingers to apply the stain to the apples of your cheeks, blending well out toward your ears.

Step 6
Do a "floating lip" with no lip liner! Use your brush to apply your lip gloss.

Step 7
Use the brush of your eyebrow gel to brush your eyebrows up and out. Fill in any gaps with the eyebrow pencil. Apply less than you think you should.

Step 8
Carefully curl your lashes and apply *one* coat of mascara, and only on the top lashes.

Step 9
Don't powder for this look! You want to have a natural glow—not a matte look. If you have oily skin, lightly powder your T-zone, which is your forehead, nose, and chin.

Why It's a Winner:

The look brings out your best features, but it's still natural enough that you can wear it anywhere.

What the Pros Say:

"Every movie star I do masters this look, because it's perfect for being 'caught' shopping with your friends or making an appearance where you just seem like you didn't have to do much to look fresh-faced and fantastic." —Joanna

The Bigger Picture:

This look *feels* like the best afternoon you ever spent hanging out and laughing with your friends. *Choose* to be that beautiful every day.

good times

The Look: This is a fun look that's a little bit more "put together." Why? It's more *monochromatic,* which means there isn't *one* feature that is drawn out. Instead, a family of colors that are less strong are used to bring the whole face together. Very hip and modern, and very, very pretty.

Tools
Toner
Tinted moisturizer with SPF
Concealer
Face/Translucent powder
Apricot crème blush
Caramel-colored lip gloss
Brow gel
Blonde eyebrow pencil
Blue-gray shimmer powder eye shadow
Lash curler
Black mascara

Get This Look

Step 1
Start with clean, prepped skin. Wash your face, then apply toner. Let the product soak into your skin for five minutes.

Step 2
Using clean hands, apply a tinted moisturizer with SPF on your face. Start at the center and blend out toward the ends of the face. Be sure to blend down your neck.

Step 3
Apply concealer with your *ring* fingertip, that's the one next to your pinkie. Dab in the bottom and top inner corners of your eyes and below your eyes, out and over, or wherever you see blue, gray, or red. Blend down and out by tapping the concealer into place until there are no distinct lines. Rub any leftover concealer on any redness around your nostrils and on any spots.

Step 4
Set your concealer by lightly tapping translucent powder over it with a puff or a fluffy brush.

Step 5
Dab just a touch of the crème blush on your fingers. Smile and swirl the crème around the apples of your cheeks. Finish by pulling the remaining product toward your ears, along the cheekbones.

Step 6
Fill in your lips with the lip gloss.

Step 7
Use the brush of your eyebrow gel to brush your eyebrows up and out. Fill in any gaps with the eyebrow pencil. Apply less than you think you should.

Step 8
Apply the blue-gray shimmer powder eye shadow to your lash line and then blend up and out to the crease, until the whole area is covered. Don't apply any shadow above the crease.

Step 9
Curl your lashes and apply *one* coat of mascara, on your top lashes only.

Why It's a Winner:

This is Piper's most exciting look. It's polished and finished. It's a very smart, in-the-know look.

What the Pros Say:

"This Gurl is a *leader*. Plus she knows how to use color to her advantage, to enhance her look of power." —Ken Pavés, celebrity hairstylist to Jessica Simpson and Eva Longoria

The Bigger Picture:

Don't wait around for another Gurl to set the trend. Try something you like and you'll be surprised how other Gurlz will respond positively and follow.

Something about Berry

The Look: Fun and fresh and bold, but not overdone; the opposite of the Gurl who's trying too hard to be beautiful. How? It blasts out *one* feature, in this case, Piper's lips. Hip and confident. Perfect for a party.

Tools
Toner
Tinted moisturizer with SPF
Concealer
Face/Translucent powder
Hot pink gloss
Brow gel
Blonde eyebrow pencil
White shimmer eye shadow
Lash curler
Black mascara

Get This Look

Step 1
Start with clean prepped skin. Wash your face, then apply toner. Let the product soak into your skin for five minutes.

Step 2
Using clean hands, apply a tinted moisturizer with SPF on your face. Start at the center and blend out toward the ends of your face. Be sure to blend down your neck.

Step 3
Apply concealer with your *ring* fingertip, that's the one next to your pinkie. Dab in the bottom and top inner corners of your eyes and below your eyes, out and over, or wherever you see blue, gray, or red. Blend down and out by tapping the concealer into place until there are no distinct lines. Rub any left-over concealer on any redness around your nostrils and on any spots.

Step 4
Set your concealer by lightly tapping face/translucent powder over the face with a puff or a fluffy brush.

Step 5
Using a lip brush, apply your gloss.

Step 6
Use the brush of your eyebrow gel to brush your eyebrows up and out. Fill in any gaps with the eyebrow pencil. Apply less than you think you should.

Step 7
Using a small eye shadow brush, apply your eye shadow along your lash line, as you would an eyeliner, from the inner corner of your eye out one third of the way, on the top and bottom.

Step 8
Curl your lashes and apply one coat of mascara, on your top lashes only. Use waterproof or smudge-proof mascara, to avoid any smudging or flaking on the white shadow, which makes it turn gray.

Why It's a Winner: This look is a total showstopper. It makes a statement. It's fun and sassy for the Glamour Gurl who's got it going on.

What the Pros Say: "This is statement makeup. It's for the Gurl who knows how to make one!" —Molly Sims, actress and supermodel

The Bigger Picture: Don't be afraid to step out of your routine. Your next great look is only one try away!

SCHLIPTIP: Where's the blush? This look doesn't use any! When you choose to accent one strong feature, tone down everything else. This look calls for bold lips, so I skipped the blush.

Tools
Toner
Tinted moisturizer with SPF
Concealer
Face/Translucent powder
Clear lip gloss
Brow gel
Blonde eyebrow pencil
Black kohl eyeliner pencil
Gray powder eye shadow
Lash curler
Black mascara

THE LOOK: This bold look is about going out and having fun. The exaggerated features are designed for night, as they are too strong for daytime.

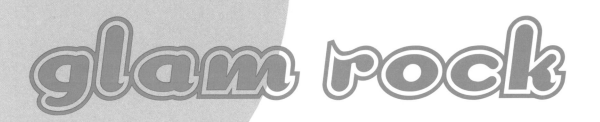

glam rock

Get This Look

Step 1
Start with clean, prepped skin. Wash your face, then apply toner. Let the product soak into your skin for five minutes.

Step 2
Using clean hands, apply a tinted moisturizer with SPF on your face. Start at the center and blend out toward the ends of the face. Be sure to blend down your neck.

Step 3
Apply concealer with your *ring* fingertip, that's the one next to your pinkie. Dab in the bottom and top inner corners of your eyes and below your eyes, out and over, or wherever you see blue, gray, or red. Blend down and out by tapping the concealer into place until there are no distinct lines. Rub any leftover concealer on any redness around your nostrils and on any spots.

Step 4
Set your concealer by lightly tapping translucent powder over it with a puff or a fluffy brush.

Step 5
Guess what? This look calls for *no* blush!

Step 6
Apply your lip gloss.

Step 7
Use the brush of your eyebrow gel to brush your eyebrows up and out. Fill in any gaps with the eyebrow pencil. Apply less than you think you should.

Step 8
To line your eyes, gently pull down your lower lid with your middle finger. Apply kohl pencil to the *inside* of your eye, from side to side. Now let go of your lid. Line your eye *below* your lashes from inside to out. Do the same *above* your lashes on the top and bottom lid.

Step 9
Dip a small eye shadow brush in gray eye shadow, flick off the excess, and apply the shadow *over* the kohl pencil above your lid. Use your eye shadow brush to smudge the kohl pencil as you go, and then begin to work the eye shadow *up* in increasingly higher side-to-side strokes across your eyelid—sort of like windshield wipers—until you reach your crease.

Step 10
Using the same technique, brush and blend shadow and kohl pencil below your eye. Don't worry if your line is not perfectly straight, as it's supposed to be a soft—not hard—line.

Step 11
Curl your lashes and apply *one* coat of mascara on your top *and* bottom lashes.

Why It's a Winner: This is a super-strong look. It says: This Gurl makes it happen. That's a really strong message. It's urban, without being too harsh. It's cool, but with class.

What the Pros Say: "I'd notice her in a crowd." —Carlos Ortiz, hairstylist to Mandy Moore

The Bigger Picture: Piper appears completely different in all four looks! So now you know with makeup you can completely change your image. Think about where you are going and how you want to present yourself before you start your application.

Carissa

This red-haired, green-eyed, gifted dancer has her eye on Broadway. The future looks bright for this Gurl!

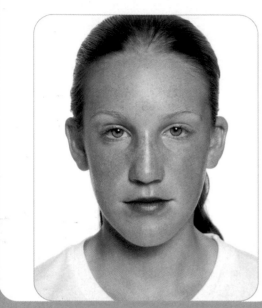

BEFORE: I lightened beneath Carissa's eyes and shaped her brow.

Tools
Toner
Tinted moisturizer with SPF
Concealer
Translucent powder
Light peach powder blush
Sheer pink lip gloss
Brow gel
Light auburn eyebrow pencil
Lash curler
Black mascara

all 4 you

The Look: *Super* natural, ideal for school or a day outdoors!

Get This Look

Step 1
Start with clean, prepped skin. Wash your face, then apply toner. Let the product soak into your skin for five minutes.

Step 2
Using clean hands, apply a tinted moisturizer with SPF on your face. Start at the center and blend out toward the ends of the face. Be sure to blend down your neck.

Step 3
Apply concealer with your *ring* fingertip, that's the one next to your pinkie. Dab in the bottom and top inner corners of your eyes and below your eyes, out and over, or wherever you see blue, gray, or red. Blend down and out by tapping the concealer into place until there are no distinct lines. Rub any leftover concealer on any redness around your nostrils and on any spots.

Step 4
Set your concealer by lightly tapping translucent powder over it with a puff or a fluffy brush.

Step 5
Lightly dust on the blush. Keep it natural.

Step 6
Sweep the lip gloss over your lips.

Step 7
Use the brush of your eyebrow gel to brush your eyebrows up and out. Fill in any gaps with the eyebrow pencil. Apply less than you think you should.

Step 8
Curl your lashes and apply one coat of mascara to both your top and bottom lashes.

SCHLIPTIP ON BLOCK: Why bother with the block? Gurl, just think of it as your skin's best friend—you'll thank me later—but only wear it during the day.

Why It's a Winner: The tones of the makeup really complement Carissa's coloring without competing with her red hair.

What the Pros Say: "Sometimes redheads have sensitive skin and it's hard to create that glow for them, but this look gives Carissa all the glow she needs." —Joanna

The Bigger Picture: The most simple looks are often the ones that make you seem the most confident!

Katie

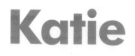

This popular little fireball can't wait for the day when she can wear makeup to school. She definitely has the gift of gab, with the biggest heart this side of Texas!

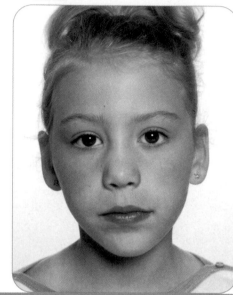

BEFORE: I choose to protect her skin with sunblock, moisturize her lips, and only brush, not tweeze, her brows.

Tools
Sunblock
Clear lip gloss
Brow gel

BABY GURL

Step 1
Start with clean, prepped skin. Wash your face and apply a sunblock. Let it soak into your skin for five minutes. Blot away any excess with a tissue.

Step 2
Swipe a bit of lip gloss over the lips.

Step 3
Use the brush of your eyebrow gel to brush your eyebrows up and out.

SCHLIPTIP: Are you breaking out all of the time? Think about your school day: Are you getting a chance to wash your face after gym class? If not, chances are that your afternoons are spent with makeup- and gym-sweat-clogged pores! Keep some oil-free makeup remover wipes in your gym bag to quickly freshen up on the way to your next class.

The Look: Clean and angelic. Perfect for a photo-op when you're not old enough to wear full-on makeup!

Why It's a Winner: Who says you have to wear makeup to look made up? In this example, a little goes a long way.

What the Pros Say: "Katie still looks her age, because her makeup is not overdone or out of place." —Joanna

The Bigger Picture: Katie's young, but she looks and acts in a way that makes her big-Gurl beautiful. Ever look back at old pictures and wonder, *how could I have worn that?* Face it: Beautiful *looks* change. Beautiful *actions* don't.

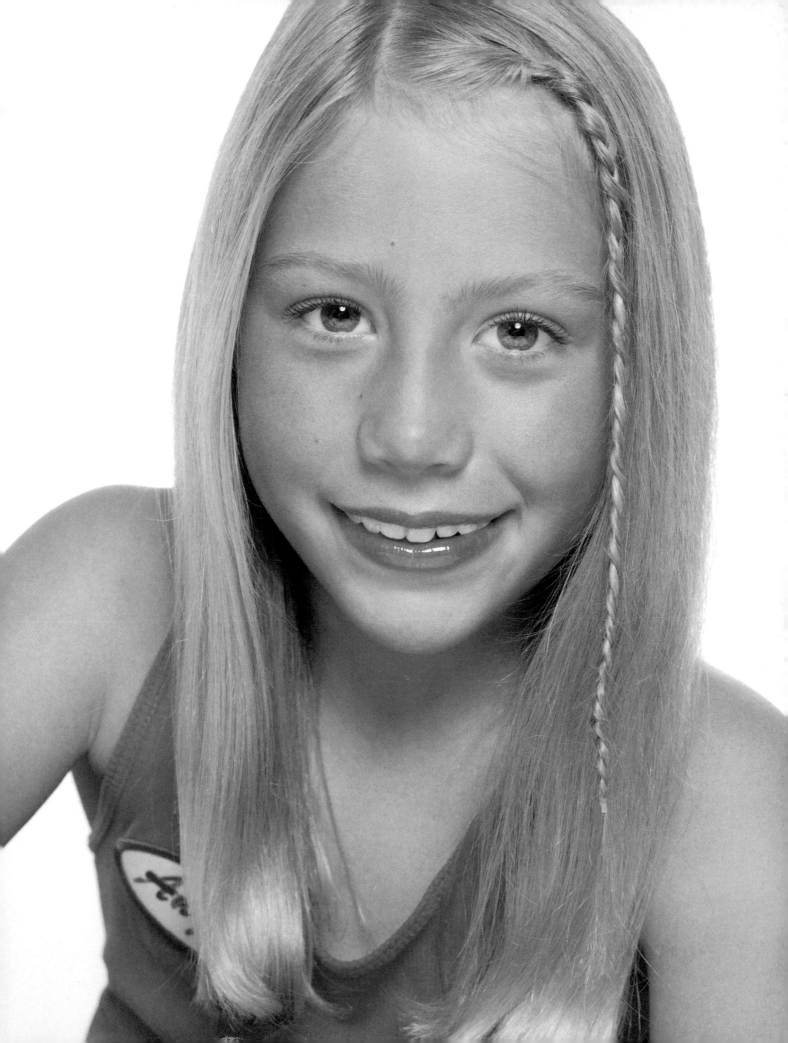

Jessica Williams
Actress

Katija Pevec
Actress

The Just for Kicks Gurlz all came together for our shoot!
Each has a unique personality, and yet they
complement one another as a team. Each Gurl

Mallory Low
Actress, Singer, and Songwriter

Francesca Catalano
Actress

took her makeup style and honored it in an individual way. They're so much fun and full of life. They have great attitudes and a lot of edge. You can tell they love what they're doing!

LIKE THIS LOOK? Same makeup on four different Gurlz = four different looks! Notice how each Gurl'z unique features and coloring stand out separately—the same technique works for them all! I also used this technique on Piper in "Skool Rules" (page 172). The change up here is bronze shimmer eye shadow and caramel lip gloss on the *Just for Kicks* Gurlz.

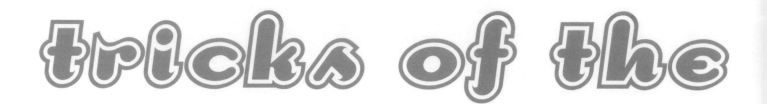

tricks of the

MAKEUP ARTIST TRICKS

Using makeup to shadow, highlight, and mask a variety of facial characteristics, makeup artists can change the way these features look in a photograph. Check out these simple tips that any Gurl can try.

WANT CHEEK BONES?
Ever notice that cheekbones are more prominent on thinner or smaller faces? Lengthen the look of your cheekbones by using a shimmery blush right on the apples of your cheeks. Then, with a large fluffy brush, *lightly* sweep a deep bronzer under your jaw line, on the sides of your face between your cheeks and ears, and down your neck. Blend back and up toward your ears. An instant slimming effect!

Every time you see a "perfect" picture in a magazine, consider how many professionals worked *for days or weeks* to create the look you see. No kidding. From the artist who did the Gurlz' makeup, to the photographer who chose the lighting and used software to alter—or *digitally retouch*—the final picture, you wouldn't believe how much a photo can change! Don't believe me? Read on for these tricks of the trade used by makeup artists and photographers.

WHAT ABOUT BLEMISHED SKIN?
To give blemished skin a smoother look, use oil-free tinted moisturizer and oil-free concealer to cover up raised blemishes. Set this makeup by dusting translucent powder all over, which will also soak up any excess oil that tends to surface in the hours after makeup application. Plus, a creamy concealer won't cake up on the flaky acne skin.

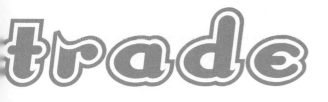

trade

NO ONE NOSE?

Forget about your nose! Play up your lashes; use a bright, shimmery blush; and swipe on a neutral lip color. Balance out any prominent facial feature by making your other features look more prominent. For example, nose too wide? Take a soft brown eye shadow and a wide shadow brush and lightly apply powder to the sides of the nose. Nose too long? Use the same soft brown shadow across the tip of your nose to "shorten" it!

BUT WHAT ABOUT A *MAJOR* MOUND?

Got a humongous mound on your face? Believe it or not, the biggest spots require the *least* concealer. Why? Piling on the product only attracts light and eyeballs. Instead, dab a small bit of *green* concealer on your blemish; this will bring down the redness. Follow up with an even smaller amount of your regular concealer, and "set" the whole thing with a *very light* dusting of loose powder. Green concealer is usually only used by the pros, so it might be harder to find, but it's well worth the search!

OR DO YOU JUST THINK YOU'RE TOO "PLAIN JANE?" THINK AGAIN!

Defy expectation! Curl your lashes and coat with mascara. Rub a little crème blush on your cheeks and lips and *presto!* It's a whole new you! In less than three minutes!

EYES WIDE OPEN!

Makeup artists use these techniques to assure a wide, bright-eyed gaze: First, use a concealer around your eyes—especially in the corners where the skin can appear dark. Set your concealer with powder, curl your lashes, and coat with mascara. Lastly, brush on a little *white* or *cream shimmer eye shadow* on the top and bottom inside corners of your eyes. Instant eye opener!

DON'T FORGET YOUR SCHOOLBAG KIT!

Always look your absolute most Glam by keeping a small bag with you, containing a crème blush stick, neutral lip gloss, tissues, and a travel-size toothbrush and toothpaste!

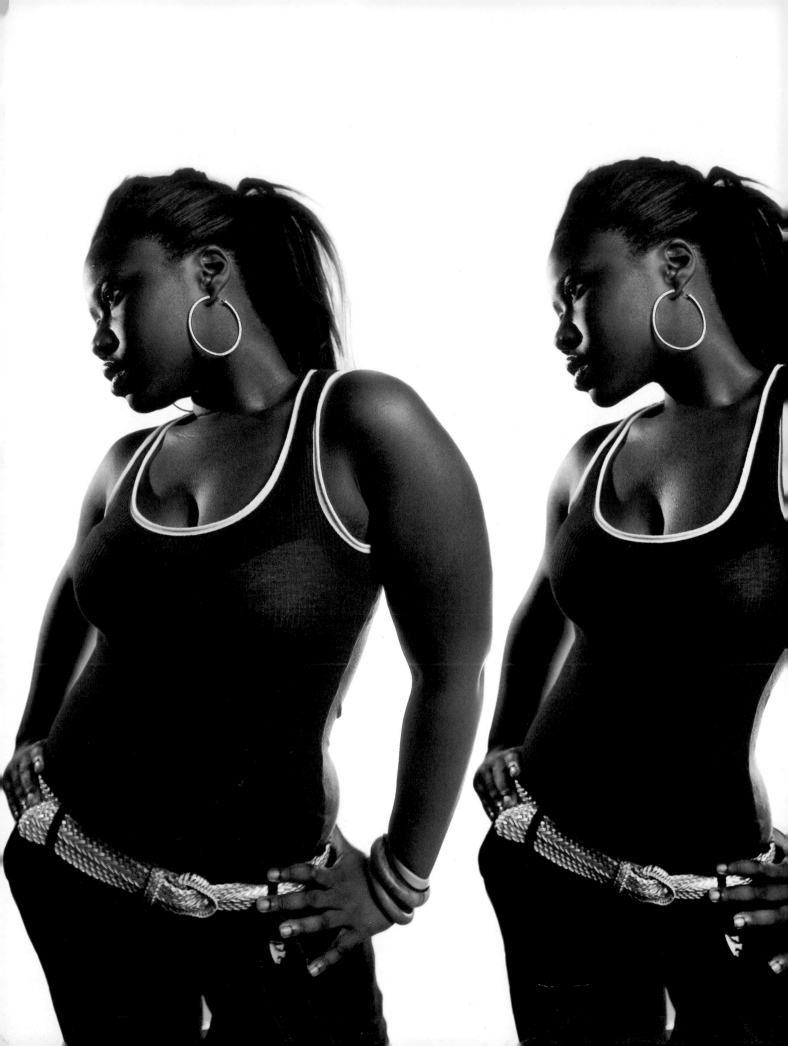

photographer and digital photography tricks

With fashion photography, what you see is not always what you get.

Many Gurlz worry that they don't look like the teen models they see. It's important for all Glamour Gurlz (even teen models!) to know that no matter how thin, pretty, or "perfect" a Gurl looks in a magazine photo, she *has* been retouched. That's because magazine fashion photography is *not supposed* to look like real life; it's an art form in itself. Sort of like the way a cartoon character is not supposed to look *exactly* like a real-life character.

Same Girl–Different Body.

So which picture is real? Photo retouching has changed all the rules. You can take red-eye out of your favorite snaps, zap a spot away, and whiten your teeth—in short, do anything you like to make an image look "perfect." In fact, almost every picture, billboard, music video, and magazine spread has been changed in some way. So if "perfect pictures" are what you want, go for it. You can retouch photos on your computer or at the photo machine at your local drugstore. But let's face it: In everyday life "perfection" simply doesn't exist. Instead, there is a great combination of different looks for different tastes.

The professional opinion? Embrace what's real about *you*—your real beauty—and play it up. As for which of these two pictures has been retouched—*you decide*. This Glamour Gurl looks beautiful in both.

two incredible photographers helped me realize this vision

a very special thanks to

Aliesh Pierce
Ali Wishneck
Alison Leslie/Marleah Leslie
  & Assoc.
Aliza Fogelson
Amy Court Kaemon
Ana Claudia Talancón
Andrea Bowen
Andre Sarmiento
Andrea Nelson Meigs/CAA
Andrew Matusik
Anne Woodward
Arielle Kebbel
Ashley Tisdale
Bill Perlman
Brandi Lord
Bren Dixie
Brie Larson
Brooke Bryant
Carlos Ortiz
Carlyne Posey
  Grager/Dramatic Artists
  Agency
Carolyn Thompson
  Goldstein/AEF
Carrie McClure/McClure PR
CeCe York/True Public
  Relations
Chad Strahan
Charnelle Smith
Christy Carlson Romano
Corey Lehmann
Crosby Carter
Darlene Reece/Sanctuary
  Group of Urban
  Management
David Michaud
Digitalretouch.net
Eileen Stringer/Howard
  Entertainment
Ellen Pompeo
Ellen Rakieten
Elizabeth Holthe
Emily Gerson Saines
Emily Urbani/Osbrink
Enzo Angileri
Erica Westheimer
Eunice Lee/CAA
Francesca Catalano

Georgie McAvenna
Gwen Kellett
Hayden Panettiere
Haylie Duff
Heather Edwards
Heather Wagner/World Music
  & Sanctuary Group
Hilary Duff
James Charles/LA Models
Jarrod Purifoy
Jeff Steele
Jennifer K. Beal
Jennifer Freeman
Jennifer Wilson
Jenny Cho
Jessica Simpson
Jessica Williams
Jewel Staite
Jill Shillaw
Jill Stewart/Creative
  Management Group
Joan Green
Jorge Insua
Justin Antony
Kate Dimmock
Katija Pevec
Ken Pavés
Kiera Chaplin
Ky Scarlet
L.A. Models
Laura Linney
Leah Buono
Leon Liu
Lesley Vogel
Lindsey Shaw
Linnea Knollmueller
Lori Rose
Luc Brinker
Madeline Leonard
Mallory Low
Mara Glauberg
Marcel Pariseau/True Public
  Relations
Maria Gagliano
Mark Soraparu/CAA
Marysarah Quinn
Meghan Wilson
Melissa Etheridge
Melissa Laskin

Mia Hansen/Aquarius PR
Michael Shaheen
Michael Tally
Michele Sydlosky
Mitch Zamarin/Asbury
  Management
Molly Sims
Monika Tashman
Nicole Nassar/Nicole Nassar
  PR
Nils Larson/Elements
  Entertainment
Pat Cutler/Cutler
  Management
Paul Marangoni
Paula Kaplan
Peter H. McGuigan
Peter Osegueda
Q'Orianka Kilcher
Robert Steinken
Samang Srisook
Sharon Lieblein
Sharon McConochie/Presse
  Public Relations
Sheryl M. Scarborough
Shinko Iura
Solange Knowles
Sophia Bush
Stella Stolper
Susan Duff
Susie Crippen
Tammy Lynn Michaels
Tara Badie
The Veronicas
Theodore Leaf
Tracy Bayne
Will Carrillo
Win Poundstone

Published in the United States by Clarkson Potter/Publishers, an imprint of the
Crown Publishing Group, a division of Random House, Inc., New York.
www.crownpublishing.com
www.clarksonpotter.com
Clarkson N. Potter is a trademark and Potter and colophon
are registered trademarks of Random House, Inc.

Special thanks to Brie Larson for permission to use
the lyrics from "Ugly" on page 150.

Photography credits appear on page 190.

Library of Congress Cataloging-in-Publication Data
Schlip, Joanna.
Glamour gurlz: the ultimate step-by-step guide to great makeup and gurl smarts / Joanna Schlip. —1st. ed.
1. Teenage girls—Health and hygiene—Juvenile literature. 2. Beauty, Personal—Juvenile literature. 3. Cosmetics—
Juvenile literature. I. Title.
RA777.25S34 2006
646.7'042—dc22   2006015139

ISBN-10: 0-307-33935-1

ISBN-13: 978-0-307-33935-5
Printed in the United States of America

Design by Jennifer K. Beal

10 9 8 7 6 5 4 3 2 1

First Edition